I0446821

Follow-up Care

and Rehabilitation

Department

The Complete Guide

ALEXANDRE CAREWELL

2

Table of Contents

« In the FCRD department, every step towards recovery is a testament to the power of human resilience and medical determination. »

Introduction

What is the FCRD service?

Follow-up and Rehabilitation Care Department, commonly referred to by the acronym FCRD, is an essential link in the patient's care pathway. Situated halfway between conventional hospitalisation and the return home, FCRD play a pivotal role in medical care, supporting patients during the crucial rehabilitation phase.

Imagine someone who has undergone major surgery or suffered a serious illness. After the acute phase of treatment, the patient is not always able to resume a normal life straight away. That's where the FCRD comes in, offering a space dedicated to both physical and psychological recovery. This service is designed to meet specific needs, particularly for patients requiring ongoing medical care, while benefiting from re-education or rehabilitation.

The FCRD is above all a global approach to health. It's not just about treating an injury or an illness, but taking the whole person into account. Multidisciplinary teams of doctors, nurses, physiotherapists, occupational therapists and other specialists work together to develop a care plan tailored to each patient. These professionals pool their expertise to ensure that each individual can regain their independence and even improve their previous quality of life.

The FCRD department is also a place to live, where patients are encouraged to play an active part in their recovery. The environment is both medicalised to ensure safety and quality of care, and warm to promote well-being. It is not simply a transition between hospital and home; it is a stage in its own right, a place where patients are rehabilitated, supported and prepared to return to their daily lives.

The FCRD embodies a holistic vision of medicine, where every stage of the healing process is taken into account, and where the patient is at the heart of everything we do. It's a world where technical care meets humanity, where clinical expertise meets empathy, and where every day, stories of resilience and rebirth are written.

Why is this book necessary?

The profession of nurse in Continuing Care and Rehabilitation (CCR) is at the croFCRDoads between advanced medical techniques and the art of human support. In the medical world, while many books are devoted to surgery, general medicine or intensive care, FCRD often remains on the sidelines, less explored, less highlighted. And yet its importance is crucial.

This book is necessary for a number of reasons:
1. Enhancing the value of an essential link in the care pathway: As an intermediary between acute hospitalisation and the return home, the FCRD plays a pivotal role in patient care. They deserve to be recognised for their true worth, not only by healthcare professionals but also by society as a whole.
2. Spotlight on an exciting profession: While many nursing students have a passing acquaintance with the FCRD, how many really know what it entails on a day-to-day basis? This book takes you into the heart of the profession, revealing its challenges, its rewards and its intrinsic richness.

3. A practical guide for professionals: Beyond theoretical knowledge, it is vital to understand the practical realities, tricks of the trade and tried and tested techniques. This book aims to fill this gap, providing practical tools to improve patient care.

4. Strengthen the community of carers: Sharing experiences, anecdotes and testimonials creates a sense of belonging. It strengthens the bond between professionals, reminding them that they are not alone in the face of daily challenges.

5. Raising awareness among the general public: For people outside the medical world, this book offers an opportunity to discover a world that is often little known. By better understanding what patients and carers in the FCRD experience, society can develop greater empathy and respect for this field.

6. Inspiration for the future: In a constantly changing medical world, it is essential to look to the future, anticipate future needs and innovate. This book is also a reflection on the potential of the FCRD, inviting us to question ourselves and to continually improve.

This book is necessary because it fills a gap, shedding light on a health sector that is too often in the shadows. It offers recognition, guidance and inspiration to all those who have anything to do with the world of Continuing Care and Rehabilitation.

Chapter 1:
THE HISTORY AND DEVELOPMENT OF FOLLOW-UP AND REHABILITATION CARE (FCRD)

Birth and development of the FCRD.

The emergence and development of follow-up and rehabilitation care (FCRD) reflects the profound changes in the healthcare system and in patients' needs over the decades. They embody an appropriate response to the growing challenges of medical care, while at the same time illustrating the constant dynamism of medicine in meeting the demands of a changing population.

Origins of FCRD
Originally, the need for post-hospital care emerged with the recognition that recovery does not end once a patient leaves hospital. In the context of the two world wars, many soldiers returned home with physical and psychological trauma. While acute medical care was essential, it soon became clear that the recovery phase required a specific approach, combining rehabilitation and psychosocial support.

Post-war developments
After the Second World War, the countries affected had to rethink their healthcare systems. It was at this time that structures dedicated to convalescence and rehabilitation began to develop, particularly in Europe. These facilities focused on rehabilitation, helping patients to regain their independence.

The rise of chronic diseases
As life expectancy increased and medical advances were made in the 20th century, chronic diseases became more prevalent. Conditions such as cardiovascular disease, diabetes and neurodegenerative disorders created a growing need for specialised post-hospital care, with rehabilitation taking centre stage.

The institutional response
Faced with these growing needs, many countries have begun to formalise and structure their FCRD services. Standards of care have been established, specialised training has been set up and dedicated funding has been allocated.

SRGs in the modern era
With the development of technology and medical advances, CRHs have incorporated cutting-edge techniques, while retaining their patient-centred approach. Telemedicine, innovative therapies and medical robotics have all found their place in modern CRHs.

Into the future
Today, the FCRD sector is at a turning point. The challenges posed by pandemics, demographic changes and medical innovations require constant adaptation. The CRHs of tomorrow will have to be even more flexible, integrative and focused on comprehensive, individualised patient care.

The FCRD have followed a fascinating path, evolving from rudimentary structures to highly specialised centres. They embody the ability of medicine to evolve in response to society's changing needs, while putting people at the heart of the therapeutic approach.

The impact of societal change and medical services in the FCRD.

Follow-up and rehabilitation care (FCRD) is at the heart of a patient's medical pathway. They act as a bridge between acute treatment and the resumption of daily life. However, like any medical field, FCRD does not operate in a vacuum. They are influenced by societal and medical changes, which over time have profoundly altered their approach and practices.

Societal changes and their impact on FCRD :
- **An ageing population:** With longer life expectancy, the number of elderly people in society is increasing. Age-related illnesses such as falls, neurodegenerative diseases and heart disease require specific rehabilitation care. FCRD have therefore had to adapt their practices and infrastructures to meet the specific needs of this age group.
- **The rise in chronic illnesses:** The prevalence of chronic illnesses, particularly diabetes, obesity and respiratory diseases, is influencing demand for CRH services. These patients require long-term care, focused on managing the disease and preventing complications.
- **Changing patient expectations: Today's** patients aspire to greater autonomy and want to be involved in their care. As a result, CRHs need to offer participatory approaches, involving patients as central players in their rehabilitation.

Medical changes and their impact on FCRD :
- **Technological advances:** The integration of new technologies, such as robotics and telerehabilitation applications, offers unprecedented opportunities for rehabilitation. These tools, which are constantly

evolving, enable more personalised and often more effective treatment.

- **Developments in rehabilitation techniques:** Medical research, based on clinical studies, has revealed new rehabilitation methods that are better adapted to certain pathologies. These discoveries have led to an updating of FCRD practices.

- **Multidisciplinary approach:** Recognising that health is not just the absence of disease, but overall well-being, the FCRD have adopted a holistic approach. This means closer collaboration between different professionals (nurses, physiotherapists, occupational therapists, psychologists, etc.) to ensure comprehensive care.

- **The challenges posed by health crises:** Events such as the COVID-19 pandemic have highlighted the need to adapt CRHs to accommodate patients with specific post-infectious needs. These crises have also highlighted the importance of responsiveness and flexibility in the management of FCRD.

As an essential link in the healthcare chain, the FCRD cannot ignore changes in society and in medicine. To remain relevant and effective, they must constantly evolve, anticipate and adapt to the new challenges posed by a changing society and a constantly evolving medical field.

Chapter 2:
UNDERSTANDING THE CENTRAL ROLE OF THE NURSE IN THE FCRD

The nurse: the pillar of the FCRD.

Nurses working in Continuing Care and Rehabilitation (CCR) are much more than just players in the care process. They are the pillar around which many interactions, care and activities revolve, enabling patients to be optimally rehabilitated. They play a central role on several fronts, and are often the first point of contact for patients and their families.

1. The nurse as care coordinator :
The specificity of FCRD lies in their multidisciplinary nature. Nurses act as liaisons between different healthcare professionals: doctors, physiotherapists, occupational therapists, psychologists and many others. They help to synchronise interventions, ensure continuity of care and guarantee comprehensive patient care.

2. The educational role :
As well as providing technical care, the FCRD nurse also has a vital educational role. They inform patients about their condition, teach them about good practice in rehabilitation and help them to understand and follow their treatment. This therapeutic education is essential if patients are to take charge of their own health.

3. Psychological support :
The rehabilitation period can be trying for the patient. Nurses, through their daily presence, are often the ones who detect signs of distress, anxiety or depression. They provide psychological support, reassurance and, if necessary, refer patients to specialists for appropriate treatment.

4. Technical expertise :
Care in the FCRD can require specific technical skills, from managing complex wounds to administering particular treatments. Nurses need to be constantly on the lookout, training regularly to meet the specific needs of their patients.

5. Prevention :
Nurses play a crucial role in preventing complications such as bedsores, hospital-acquired infections and thrombosis. Thanks to their meticulous observation and in-depth knowledge of the patient, they are often the first to identify the warning signs of complications and act accordingly.

6. The human dimension :
Through their daily contact with patients, nurses establish a relationship of trust, which is essential to the success of the rehabilitation process. It is often with them that patients share their hopes, fears and difficulties. The nurse provides a sympathetic ear, empathy and support that go well beyond technical care.

The FCRD nurse is the cornerstone of care. They ensure continuity of care, guarantee the quality of care and establish that all-important relationship with the patient that often makes all the difference in the rehabilitation process. Without them, the FCRD could not function with such efficiency and humanity.

Differences and similarities with other departments.

Follow-up and rehabilitation care (FCRD) has its own characteristics that distinguish it from many other hospital services. However, they also share a number of similarities with the latter, as they form part of a continuum of care. To fully understand their unique place in the medical landscape, it is relevant to compare them with other services, such as acute care, intensive care and long-term care units.

Differences between FCRD and other services :
- **Nature of care:** FCRD focus mainly on rehabilitation, while acute and intensive care focus on the treatment of serious medical conditions or emergencies.
- **Length of stay:** stays in FCRD tend to be longer than in acute care departments, but shorter than in long-term care units. Their aim is to prepare patients to return home or to another less medical environment.
- **Multidisciplinary approach:** Although all hospital departments work as a team, the multidisciplinary approach is particularly pronounced in the FCRD. This service often involves a variety of specialists, such as physiotherapists, occupational therapists, speech therapists, etc.
- **Infrastructure and equipment:** FCRD often have specific equipment and infrastructure for rehabilitation, such as physiotherapy rooms or therapeutic swimming pools.

Similarities between FCRD and other services :
- **Patient at the centre: Whatever** the service, the patient's well-being is always at the heart of our concerns. Every professional strives to provide quality care to meet the patient's needs.
- **Coordination of care:** In all departments, it is essential to ensure effective coordination between the various health professionals in order to guarantee optimal care.
- **Continuum of care:** The FCRD, like other services, is part of a care pathway. A patient may move from intensive care to acute care, then to the FCRD, before eventually being transferred to a long-term care unit.

- **Continuing education:** In all departments, healthcare professionals, including nurses, need to keep their knowledge and skills up to date in order to provide the best possible care.
- **Administrative and regulatory   challenges:** Like all hospital services, FCRD face funding, regulatory and management challenges.

FCRD occupy a special place in the hospital landscape. While they share a number of similarities with other services, they are distinctly different in that they focus on rehabilitation and preparing patients to return to a less medical environment.

The importance of multidisciplinarity.

Multidisciplinarity is an essential concept in medicine, relying on the collaboration of professionals from different disciplines to provide comprehensive and coherent care for the patient. In the world of healthcare, where each speciality holds a piece of the vast body of medical knowledge, the multidisciplinary approach is not only a necessity, but also a strength.

Imagine the journey of a patient in Continuing Care and Rehabilitation (CCR) after a cerebrovascular accident (CVA). Recovery does not depend solely on medication or surgery, but on a multitude of interventions. Occupational therapists work on restoring everyday movement, physiotherapists on mobility and muscle strength, speech therapists on any speech problems, and nurses on coordinating care and preventing complications. Each of these professionals contributes essential expertise, but it is their harmonious and complementary work together that will enable patients to regain their independence.

This collaboration is not just a combination of interventions. It also promotes fluid communication between professionals, ensuring that every medical decision is informed and adapted to the patient's overall context. For example, a change in drug treatment may affect the rehabilitation programme, or an observation made by the physiotherapist may influence nursing care. Thanks to our multi-disciplinary approach, these interactions take place with mutual transparency and understanding.

In addition to the medical benefits, the multidisciplinary approach also enriches the patient-professional relationship. Patients feel supported, listened to and considered as a whole, with responses tailored to their physical and psychological concerns. Complementary skills ensure comprehensive care, where every aspect of the patient's health is taken into account.

Multidisciplinarity is much more than a working method; it is a philosophy of care. It reflects the recognition that, in the medical field, the pooling of knowledge and skills is the guarantee of optimal care, focused on the patient's well-being and recovery.

Chapter 3:
ADMISSION TO THE FCRD

The admission process:
from application to installation.

The process of admission to Continuing Care and Rehabilitation (CCR) is a crucial stage, orchestrating the patient's transition from one medical environment to another, with the aim of rehabilitation and gradual reintegration. Although this transition may seem administrative, it is essential to ensure continuity and quality of care. From the admission request to the patient's arrival on the ward, every step is designed to ensure the patient's safety and well-being.

It usually starts with a medical recommendation. Whether it is from a GP, a surgeon following an operation or a specialist in an acute care department, the need for rehabilitation is identified. The doctor then draws up a request for admission to the FCRD, detailing the medical context, the specific rehabilitation needs and the objectives to be achieved.

This request is then assessed by the FCRD team, often led by a rehabilitation doctor. The latter examines the patient's medical records, assesses the relevance of the admission in terms of the department's capacity and specialities, and checks the availability of places. This ensures that the department can adequately meet the patient's needs.

Once the application has been accepted, the administrative process begins. The patient's contact details, health insurance and other relevant details are collected. This phase, although bureaucratic, is vital to ensure that the patient is cared for smoothly and without hindrance throughout their stay.

As the date of admission approaches, communication is established with the patient and their family. They are given practical information, such as things to bring with them, visiting times and accommodation arrangements. This stage prepares patients for their arrival, reassuring them and answering any questions they may have.

Finally, on the day of admission, the patient is welcomed by the FCRD team. After the admission formalities, an initial medical assessment is carried out to establish a personalised care plan. The nurse, who is key to this transition, takes the time to settle the patient in, familiarise them with their new environment and introduce them to the medical team.

The admission process, although it may seem linear, is in fact the reflection of constant attention paid to the patient. From the first referral to settling into their room, each stage is designed to ensure that patients feel cared for, listened to and confident, thus starting their rehabilitation journey in the best possible conditions.

Initial assessment of the patient.

The initial assessment of a patient in Continuing Care and Rehabilitation (CCR) is a fundamental stage that lays the foundations for the entire rehabilitation process. It enables a complete medical and functional assessment to be carried out, and the patient's specific needs to be identified. This assessment guides the development of an individualised care plan, focused on rehabilitation objectives.

As soon as the patient arrives, the assessment begins with a **medical interview** with the rehabilitation doctor. During this discussion, the patient's medical history is taken, i.e. all the information about their medical and surgical history and the circumstances that led to their admission to the FCRD. The patient's complaints and expectations are also explored, giving an overall view of his situation.

The **systems review** is then carried out. This involves questioning the patient about each body system (cardiovascular, respiratory, digestive, etc.) to detect any symptoms or anomalies.

The **physical examination phase** follows. The doctor carries out an overall assessment, reviewing the various bodily functions. For example, he assesses muscle strength, joint mobility, sensitivity and balance.

Alongside the medical assessment, other professionals are involved:
- The **occupational therapist** assesses the patient's ability to carry out activities of daily living, such as dressing, eating and managing personal care.
- The **physiotherapist** examines motor function, gait quality and respiratory capacity.
- If necessary, the **speech therapist will** assess any speech, swallowing or cognitive disorders.
- **Psychologists** or neuropsychologists may be called in to explore the patient's emotional state and resilience, or to assess any cognitive problems.
- The **nurse** plays a cross-disciplinary role, gathering information on the patient's experiences, habits, level of autonomy, medication and any therapeutic education needs.

All this data, meticulously collected, is then compiled into a **care plan**. This will be regularly reassessed and adjusted according to the patient's progress.

The initial assessment of a patient in an FCRD is therefore a multi-dimensional process, involving a multi-disciplinary team. It lays the foundations for holistic, patient-centred care aimed at helping patients regain their independence.

The crucial role of the nurse in coordination of care on admission.

As a front-line healthcare professional, nurses play a pivotal role when patients are admitted to the Continuing Care and Rehabilitation Unit (CCRU). At the croFCRDoads between medicine, organisation and the human dimension of care, nurses are often the first face patients meet and the last they see at the end of the day. In this context, coordinating care on admission is a major responsibility for nurses, and here's how it works in practice.

1. First point of contact and initial assessment :
When patients arrive at the FCRD, it is usually the nurse who receives them, offers them an initial orientation and carries out an initial assessment. This assessment, although more focused on nursing care, complements the doctor's assessment by shedding light on the patient's general condition, immediate needs and concerns.

2. Communication with the multidisciplinary team :
The nurse gathers essential information that will be shared with the entire care team: doctors, physiotherapists, occupational therapists, psychologists, etc. They make sure that everyone is aware of the patient's particular needs, whether they be allergies to medication, dietary restrictions or specific psychological requirements.

3. Organisation of immediate care :

Depending on the patient's condition on arrival, immediate care may be required. The nurse coordinates these interventions, whether they involve administering medication, applying dressings or putting the patient on oxygen therapy.

4. Patient education and reassurance :

Admission can be a source of stress for patients. The nurse takes the time to explain procedures, introduce the care team and answer any questions. This reassures the patient and facilitates their integration into the department.

5. Coordination with external services :

If the patient requires further tests, the nurse coordinates these with the relevant departments, whether imaging, laboratory or specialist consultations.

6. Planning the care plan :

In collaboration with the medical team, the nurse draws up a care plan for the patient. This plan takes into account the patient's medical needs, rehabilitation goals and preferences.

7. Transmission of information :

As the nurses work in shifts, it is essential that information is transmitted clearly and accurately between the day and night teams, thus ensuring continuity of care.

The nurse, by virtue of his central position and proximity to the patient, is an essential link in the coordination of care on admission to the FCRD. They ensure the smooth running of interventions, patient safety and help to establish a relationship of trust, the cornerstone of successful care.

Chapter 4:
TECHNIQUES AND
SPECIFIC SKILLS IN FCRD

Medical skills specific to the FCRD.

Follow-up and rehabilitation care (FCRD) is a crucial stage in a patient's care. Its aim is to restore impaired function, optimise independence and prepare patients for their return home or to a suitable facility. This mission requires healthcare professionals to have specific skills, adapted to the complexity of the needs of the patients under their care.

1. Functional assessment skills :
FCRD professionals must be able to assess patients' functional capacity. This means mastering the tools and techniques needed to assess muscle strength, joint mobility, balance and coordination.

2. Rehabilitation expertise :
Rehabilitation is at the heart of FCRD. Caregivers must therefore have advanced skills in physiotherapy, occupational therapy, speech therapy, etc., depending on their respective specialities.

3. Knowledge of common pathologies:
FCRD patients often come after acute care hospitalisations for various pathologies such as stroke, trauma or major surgery. A thorough understanding of these pathologies and their implications is essential.

4. Pain management :
Patients undergoing rehabilitation may suffer from chronic or acute pain. FCRD carers need to be trained in pain management, using both medicinal and non-medicinal approaches.

5. Psychosocial skills :
Rehabilitation is not just physical. FCRD professionals must be able to assess and support patients' emotional, psychological and social needs, helping them to overcome the obstacles associated with their illness or condition.

6. Interdisciplinary coordination and communication :
The FCRD is a highly collaborative environment. Caregivers must therefore excel at communicating with other healthcare professionals (doctors, nurses, therapists) to ensure coherent and comprehensive care.

7. Therapeutic education :
One of the roles of the FCRD is to prepare patients for their return home. This often involves educating patients (and sometimes their families) about their condition, treatments, what to do or not to do, and the adaptations needed for daily life.

8. Expertise in medical technologies :
Technological advances have meant that a wide range of modern tools and equipment have been incorporated into FCRD care, including mobilisation equipment, virtual reality technologies for rehabilitation and medical monitoring devices.

9. Holistic approach :
In FCRD, the patient is considered as a whole. This requires an ability to integrate all facets of an individual's health: physical, emotional, social and cognitive.

10. Adaptability :
Finally, every patient is unique, and rehabilitation can present unexpected challenges. The ability to adapt, innovate and adjust care plans is an essential skill in CRH.

The specificity of the FCRD lies in this combination of medical expertise, rehabilitation skills and a patient-centred approach, offering personalised, multi-dimensional care.

Pain management and advanced care techniques.

Pain management is a key issue in follow-up and rehabilitation care. Many patients suffer from pain following surgery, trauma or chronic illness. Appropriate pain management is essential for the patient's comfort and well-being, but also to promote rehabilitation. Combining this management with advanced care techniques offers a modern, holistic approach to treatment.

1. Pain assessment :
Above all, it is crucial to assess pain correctly. Scales such as the visual analogue scale (VAS) or the numerical scale are commonly used. This assessment takes into account the intensity, location, nature (acute vs. chronic pain) and impact of the pain on quality of life.

2. Pharmacological approaches :
- **Analgesics**: These range from simple analgesics (paracetamol) to opiates (morphine), depending on the severity of the pain.
- **Non-steroidal anti-inflammatory drugs (NSAIDs):** Useful for pain of inflammatory origin.
- **Antidepressants and anticonvulsants**: These drugs can be effective, particularly for neuropathic pain.

3. Advanced pain management techniques :
- **Transcutaneous Neurostimulation (TENS)**: A technique which uses small electrical currents to stimulate the nerves and thus reduce the perception of pain.
- **Nerve block**: Injections of medication to temporarily block a group of nerves and relieve pain.
- **Analgesic pump**: Device for the controlled administration of opiates directly into the nervous system.

4. Non-pharmacological approaches :

- **Physiotherapy**: Specific movements can help relieve pain and improve mobility and strength.
- **Thermotherapy and cryotherapy**: The use of heat or cold can have analgesic effects.
- **Acupuncture**: This age-old Chinese technique can bring significant relief to some patients.
- **Manual therapies**: Like osteopathy or chiropractic, they can be beneficial for musculoskeletal pain.

5. Psychological approaches :

- **Cognitive behavioural therapy (CBT)**: This helps patients to manage pain by changing the way they perceive and react to it.
- **Relaxation and meditation**: Techniques that can help relax the body and mind, reducing the perception of pain.

6. Innovative technologies :

- **Virtual reality**: Studies show that virtual reality can help distract the mind from pain, providing a kind of 'cognitive' analgesia.
- **Biofeedback:** Technique that teaches patients how to control physiological functions to improve their state of health.

7. Therapeutic education :

It is essential to teach patients to understand their pain, to express it and to use techniques to relieve it, but also to avoid behaviour that could make it worse.

Pain management in the FCRD is based on a multimodal approach, combining traditional techniques with modern innovations. It requires close collaboration between the patient, nurses, doctors and therapists, always with the aim of offering the patient the best possible quality of life.

Mobilisation techniques and early rehabilitation.

Mobilisation and early rehabilitation techniques play an essential role in Continuing Care and Rehabilitation (CCR). These approaches aim to promote movement, minimise physical deconditioning and facilitate a return to independence. Starting rehabilitation early, even in acute conditions, can reduce secondary complications and optimise recovery. Let's take a closer look.

1. The importance of early mobilisation :
Early mobilisation helps prevent complications associated with prolonged immobility, such as muscle atrophy, deep vein thrombosis, pneumonia and bedsores. It also helps improve blood circulation and maintain muscle mass.

2. Passive mobilisation techniques :
Used when the patient cannot move independently, they involve the use of devices or the intervention of a carer to move the patient's limbs. These techniques may include range-of-motion exercises or the use of devices such as cycle ergometers for the lower limbs.

3. Active assisted mobilisation :
The patient actively participates but receives assistance. For example, a physiotherapist can support the weight of a limb while helping the patient to move.

4. Active mobilisation :
The patient performs movements on their own. This may involve bed exercises, transferring from bed to chair, or strengthening and balance exercises.

5. Techniques specific to early rehabilitation :
- **Getting out of bed early**: Encourage the patient to sit up and get out of bed as soon as possible.
- **Assisted walking**: The use of walkers or crutches to help patients regain their ability to walk.

- **Breathing exercises**: These improve lung function, particularly after thoracic or abdominal surgery.

6. Early rehabilitation specific to the condition :

Depending on the medical condition, techniques may vary:
- For a stroke: work on mobility, coordination, speech and swallowing.
- After orthopaedic surgery: early movement of the affected joint, muscle strengthening and work on range of movement.

7. The importance of psychological support :

Early rehabilitation is not limited to the physical dimension. Psychological support is essential to help patients overcome mental and emotional barriers, and to reinforce their motivation to participate actively in rehabilitation.

8. Technology and rehabilitation :

Modern tools such as virtual reality, exoskeletons or biofeedback platforms can be integrated to improve rehabilitation outcomes and make the process more engaging for the patient.

The key to successful mobilisation and early rehabilitation lies in an individualised, interdisciplinary approach involving doctors, nurses, physiotherapists, occupational therapists and other professionals. The aim is not only to restore function, but also to give patients the tools and confidence to return to an active, independent life.

Chapter 5:
DAILY CHALLENGES
AND HOW TO OVERCOME THEM

Managing complex situations :
the recalcitrant patient
difficult family circumstances.

Follow-up and rehabilitation care (FCRD) often lies at the intersection of medicine, psychology and social care. As a result, nurses in FCRD are regularly faced with complex situations. Whether it's a recalcitrant patient, a difficult life history, or a tense family context, each situation requires particular finesse, patience and skill if it is to be managed effectively.

1. The recalcitrant patient :
The patient who refuses or resists treatment can be one of the greatest challenges. This refusal may be due to fear, mistrust, depression or other psychological factors.
- **Establishing a relationship of trust**: taking the time to listen, express empathy and reassure the patient.
- **Understand the source of the recalcitrance**: is it a fear of pain, a lack of understanding of the treatment, or something else?
- **Involving specialists**: A psychologist or social worker can contribute their expertise to the patient's care.

2. Difficult family background :
The family environment plays a crucial role in a patient's recovery. However, not all families are supportive or understanding.
- **Organise family** meetings: These provide an opportunity to discuss concerns, offer education and

clarify each member's role in the rehabilitation process.

- **Conflict mediation**: In tense situations, mediation can help resolve disagreements and establish constructive communication.
- **Outside support**: Sometimes it may be necessary to call on social services or associations to provide additional support for the family.

3. Managing difficult life histories :

Past trauma, whether physical or psychological, can influence the way a patient responds to treatment.

- **Specialist training**: Ensuring that staff are trained to recognise and manage signs of trauma.
- **Patient-centred approach**: Adapting the treatment plan to the patient's specific needs and concerns.
- **Working with mental health specialists**: In some cases, the support of a psychologist or psychiatrist can be beneficial.

4. Team communication :

Fluid communication between all members of the care team is essential to ensure optimal care.

- **Regular meetings**: These are an opportunity to share information, discuss challenges and coordinate actions.
- **Ongoing training**: Organise training sessions on managing complex situations to enhance the team's skills.

Managing complex situations in the FCRD requires a multidimensional approach that goes well beyond medical care. Nurses, as the backbone of this service, play a crucial role, often being the first line of interaction with patients and their families. With empathy, patience, skill and collaboration, they can navigate through these challenges to ensure the well-being and recovery of their patients.

The emotional and psychological challenges of rehabilitation.

Rehabilitation, although focused on physical recovery, inevitably involves the patient's emotional and psychological dimensions. The healing process is not limited to wound healing or muscle re-education; it also involves regaining autonomy, managing pain, accepting new bodily realities and adapting to a new state of normality.

1. Confronting a new reality :
When a patient enters rehabilitation, they may be faced with the realisation that their life may never be the same. This reality may give rise to feelings of disbelief, denial, anger or grief for the life they knew before.

2. Uncertainty and anxiety :
Not knowing what to expect, how long rehabilitation will last, or to what extent recovery will be complete can be a major source of stress for the patient.

3. The challenges of chronic pain :
Pain, particularly when it is persistent, can have devastating effects on morale and psychological well-being. It can lead to feelings of despair, irritability and even depression.

4. Difficulties of acceptance :
Accepting body changes, such as the loss of a limb or the presence of a major scar, requires considerable psychological adjustment. Acceptance is a process that can take time and psychological support.

5. The challenges of independence and autonomy :
Loss of autonomy, even temporarily, can have a profound effect on a patient's self-esteem and sense of dignity.

6. Reactions of family and friends :
The way in which family and friends react to the situation can influence the patient's emotional well-being. Support, or the lack of it, can have a significant impact on the rehabilitation process.

7. The challenges of resuming daily activities :
Resuming simple tasks, such as dressing or feeding oneself, can be a source of frustration, particularly when it comes to rediscovering how to perform these once-familiar actions.

8. Fears of recidivism or deterioration :
For some conditions, the fear of a relapse or worsening of the condition may haunt the patient.
Faced with these emotional and psychological challenges, it is essential to offer appropriate psychological support throughout the rehabilitation process. This can take the form of psychotherapy sessions, support groups, art or music therapy workshops, or social work.

Each patient is unique, as is their rehabilitation journey. Understanding and responding to these emotional and psychological challenges is an essential part of ensuring comprehensive and holistic rehabilitation.

How to maintain balance between empathy and professionalism.

In the medical world, and particularly in the context of Continuing and Rehabilitation Care (CRT), maintaining a balance between empathy and professionalism is a major challenge for nurses and other healthcare professionals. Every patient is an individual with their own story, their own pain and their own hopes. Connecting with them emotionally can improve care, but it is also crucial to maintain a certain distance to ensure quality of care and protect the mental health of the carer.

1. Recognising the value of empathy :
Empathy, the ability to understand and feel what others are going through, is fundamental to the relationship between carer and patient. It fosters trust, facilitates communication and improves adherence to treatment.

2. Establish clear limits :
While it is essential to show empathy, healthcare professionals must also set clear boundaries to protect their own mental health. This could mean not giving out their personal phone number, not accepting friends on social networks or not getting involved in the patient's personal affairs.

3. Do not pass judgement :
A professional must treat each patient with respect, regardless of their background, beliefs or behaviour. Avoiding judgement fosters an authentic and empathetic relationship.

4. Training in therapeutic communication :
Specific techniques, such as active listening and reformulation, enable you to show empathy while remaining professional. These techniques can be developed through specific training courses.

5. Knowing how to disconnect :
After a day's work, especially if it's been emotionally charged, it's crucial to find ways to disconnect. This can involve relaxing activities, sport, meditation or simply spending time with loved ones.

6. Using supervision or debriefing :
Regular supervision or debriefing with colleagues or supervisors can help you manage the emotions you feel at work. It's an opportunity to express your feelings, receive advice and reflect on your practice.

7. Remember the role of the carer :

The primary role of the carer is to provide quality medical care. While empathy is essential to understanding the patient's emotional needs, it is equally crucial not to let these emotions overwhelm the primary role.

8. Protecting yourself :

Healthcare professionals are also vulnerable to burnout, depression and other mental health problems. Being aware of your own needs and putting prevention strategies in place are essential to maintaining the balance between empathy and professionalism.

Finally, being an empathetic and professional carer requires constant work on oneself, reflection on one's practice and the implementation of strategies to protect one's mental health while offering quality care.

Chapter 6:
WORKING AS PART OF AN FCRD TEAM

The importance of communication between healthcare professionals.

Communication between healthcare professionals is one of the pillars of the healthcare system. It ensures that patients receive the best possible overall care, promotes a better understanding of medical issues and reduces the risk of errors or misunderstandings. Let's look at why this communication is so fundamental.

Harmonisation of care :
Caring for a patient often requires the involvement of several health professionals: doctors, nurses, Caregivers, physiotherapists, psychologists, etc. Fluid communication helps to harmonise care, ensure continuity of care and avoid contradictory or redundant actions.

Reducing medical errors:
Poor communication is one of the main causes of medical errors. By communicating regularly and clearly, professionals can keep each other informed about current treatments, allergies, medical history or any other element crucial to patient safety.

Facilitating the transmission of information :
Handover, written transmissions, multidisciplinary meetings... these are all key moments when communication plays a major role. Missed or misinterpreted information can have a major impact on the quality of care.

Time optimisation :
Effective communication avoids duplication, unnecessary examinations and contradictory actions. It allows care to be better organised, optimising everyone's time.

Improving well-being at work :
Good communication strengthens team cohesion, reduces tension and prevents conflict. Working in an environment where you feel listened to and where information flows freely helps to improve well-being at work.

Adapting to medical developments :
Medicine is constantly evolving. Protocols change, new treatments appear and recommendations are regularly updated. Effective communication allows this new information to be disseminated quickly, ensuring that everyone's knowledge is kept up to date.

Understanding psychosocial issues :
A patient is not just a diagnosis or a list of symptoms. They come with their own history, concerns and fears. By communicating with each other, professionals can better understand these psychosocial issues, which are essential for comprehensive care.

Facilitating multidisciplinary care :
Many patients require multidisciplinary care. Communication between the various professionals enables this care to be coordinated, objectives to be harmonised and continuity of follow-up to be ensured.

Communication between healthcare professionals is essential to guarantee the safety, efficiency and quality of care. However, to be fully effective, it requires skills, appropriate training and suitable tools.

Working with doctors, physiotherapists and occupational therapists and other team members.

Collaboration between the various members of the medical team is essential to guarantee comprehensive, coordinated patient care. Each professional brings a unique and complementary expertise, creating a synergy that benefits the patient. Let's explore how this collaboration works between nurses, doctors, physiotherapists, occupational therapists and other members of the team.

1. With doctors :
Nurses work closely with doctors. They are often the first to observe changes in the patient's condition and can therefore provide valuable information to the doctor. Together, they discuss treatment plans, medication and the patient's specific needs. The nurse also carries out the doctor's prescriptions, while acting as a link between the patient and the doctor.

2. With physiotherapists :
The role of the physiotherapist is to work on the patient's mobility and functionality. The nurse and physiotherapist often work together to identify mobilisation needs, potential contraindications to certain movements and the best way to support the patient's rehabilitation.

3. With occupational therapists :
The occupational therapist focuses on daily activities and the patient's ability to function independently. The nurse may work with the occupational therapist to share observations about the patient's abilities, help adapt the patient's environment to facilitate independence and support the occupational therapist's interventions.

4. With other team members :
In addition to these professionals, the team may also include psychologists, dieticians and social workers, among others. Nurses play a central role in this team, as they are often in direct and continuous contact with the patient. They can provide essential information to each member of the team and help coordinate care.

5. Communication :
The key to this collaboration is open and regular communication. This can take the form of team meetings,

medical notes, oral transmissions or any other means of sharing essential information.

6. Continuing education :

Ongoing training enables professionals to understand each other's roles and responsibilities. It can also help to develop inter-professional skills, fostering better collaboration.

7. Mutual respect :

Each professional brings unique expertise to the table. Recognising and valuing this expertise fosters healthy and productive collaboration. Mutual respect is the foundation of an effective team.

8. Common objectives :

Although each professional has his or her own areas of expertise, the ultimate goal is always the patient's health and well-being. Keeping this objective in mind helps to overcome any disagreements or misunderstandings.

Collaboration between the different members of the medical team is essential to provide comprehensive, coordinated care. This requires communication, mutual respect and commitment to common goals.

Coordination techniques and care planning.

Coordinating and planning care is crucial to ensuring that patients receive comprehensive, effective care. They enable the interventions of each professional to be harmonised, respond appropriately to the patient's needs and optimise the resources available. This approach requires both clinical expertise and management skills.

1. Initial assessment :

Before any planning, it is essential to carry out a full assessment of the patient. This must include medical, psychosocial and functional aspects. This assessment will enable priority needs and care objectives to be identified.

2. Drawing up a care plan :
Based on the assessment, a care plan is drawn up. This details the interventions to be carried out, the professionals involved, the objectives to be achieved and the timetable for implementation. This plan must be flexible to adapt to changes in the patient's condition.

3. Communication :
Coordination requires fluid communication between the various players involved. Multidisciplinary meetings, written and oral communications and digital tools are all ways of ensuring good communication.

4. Monitoring and reassessment :
The patient's situation must be regularly reassessed in order to adjust the care plan accordingly. These reassessments can be scheduled or carried out according to the changes observed.

5. Involving patients and their families :
Care coordination is all the more effective when patients and their families are involved. They can provide essential information, participate in decision-making and contribute to the implementation of the care plan.

6. Use of coordination tools :
There are a number of tools that can facilitate coordination, such as shared medical records, scheduling software, monitoring applications, and so on. These tools centralise information, facilitate communication and ensure rigorous monitoring.

7. Further training :
Coordination techniques evolve over time, as do patient needs and available resources. Regular training is therefore essential to keep up to date and optimise your practices.

8. Consideration of available resources :
Planning must be adapted to the resources available (staff, equipment, time). This sometimes means prioritising certain actions or looking for alternative solutions.

9. Collaboration with external structures :
In some cases, the patient may require external assistance (hospitalisation at home, social services, etc.). Coordination with these structures is essential to ensure continuity of care.

10. Documentation :
All interventions, assessments and decisions must be rigorously documented. This guarantees traceability of care, facilitates communication and helps to ensure the quality and safety of interventions.

Care coordination and planning are dynamic, patient-centred processes that require close collaboration between the various professionals and constant adaptation to the needs and resources available.

Chapter 7:
TECHNOLOGICAL TOOLS IN FCRD

Technological developments and its impact on FCRD.

Technological developments have profoundly altered the landscape of Continuing Care and Rehabilitation (CCR). These advances have introduced new methods, tools and approaches to the treatment and care of patients, making care more effective and changing the way professionals work. Let's tackle this impact in a fluid and coherent way.

The digital revolution has brought about an unprecedented transformation in the medical sector. In the context of FCRD, several key elements of this technological evolution deserve to be highlighted.

1. Telemedicine :
Telemedicine has opened the door to remote consultation, enabling patients to benefit from medical expertise without having to travel. For FCRD, this means better access to specialists, easier post-hospital follow-up and improved continuity of care, particularly for patients who are far away or have reduced mobility.

2. Robotics and assistive devices :
Robotic innovations have led to the introduction of exoskeletons, mobilisation robots and other assistive devices. These tools, used in rehabilitation, support and reinforce patients' movements, speeding up their recovery and optimising their rehabilitation.

3. Virtual and augmented reality :
Virtual and augmented reality offer stimulating and controlled environments for rehabilitation. Patients can, for example, practise walking or gripping in virtual scenarios

adapted to their needs, while benefiting from real-time feedback.

4. Medical information systems :
Electronic medical records and digital patient management platforms have led to improved traceability, greater access to information and enhanced coordination between professionals. These systems contribute to more personalised and better-informed care.

5. Remote monitoring devices :
Thanks to connected devices, it is now possible to monitor certain patient health parameters in real time, such as heart rate, blood pressure and activity levels. This makes it possible to adjust care and interventions according to actual needs, and to anticipate certain complications.

6. Training and simulation :
New technologies also offer training opportunities. Medical simulators, for example, allow professionals to train and perfect their skills in conditions that are close to the real thing, but without any risk to the patient.

The impact of these technological developments on nursing homes is undeniable. They offer opportunities to improve the quality of care, optimise rehabilitation and make life easier for professionals. However, they also raise challenges, particularly in terms of adaptation, training and ethics. It is essential that these innovations are integrated in a considered way, always putting the patient at the heart of the process.

Appliances and tools
modern rehabilitation centres.

The world of rehabilitation has undergone a remarkable evolution thanks to the introduction of modern equipment and tools. These innovations have been designed to facilitate recovery, improve functional capabilities and support healthcare professionals in their mission. Let's take a closer look at some of these devices and tools, which are now essential in Continuing Care and Rehabilitation (CCR) departments.

1. Exoskeletons :
These robotic structures are worn on the body to assist or amplify movement. They are particularly useful for re-educating patients with muscular weakness or mobility problems.

2. Virtual reality platforms :
Virtual reality programmes are used to immerse patients in a stimulating environment, where they can practise specific rehabilitation exercises, while receiving real-time feedback on their performance.

3. Treadmills with body weight support :
These treadmills, fitted with a harness, allow patients to walk without carrying their full body weight, facilitating rehabilitation after certain injuries or surgical procedures.

4. Biofeedback devices :
These tools provide visual or audio feedback on muscle activity or other bodily functions, helping patients to better understand and control their own bodies during rehabilitation.

5. Laser therapy :
Used to treat pain and inflammation and accelerate tissue healing, laser therapy is a non-invasive procedure that often complements other rehabilitation methods.

6. Tables and traction equipment :
These devices are designed to stretch certain parts of the body, particularly the spine, to reduce pain and improve mobility.

7. Electrotherapy equipment :
Using electrical impulses to stimulate muscles or alleviate pain, these devices are commonly used to treat various muscle and nerve disorders.

8. Robots for limb rehabilitation :
These robots assist or guide the movements of the upper or lower limbs, providing targeted, tailored rehabilitation.

9. Therapy balls and rollers :
Although simple, these tools are essential for physiotherapy, helping to improve flexibility, strength and coordination.

10. Mobile applications and wearables :
Connected watches, sensors and dedicated applications can track physical activity, posture, sleep and other parameters, providing valuable information for the rehabilitation process.

These modern devices and tools, combined with proven therapeutic approaches, enable more personalised, effective and engaging care for patients in the CRH. As technology continues to evolve, it is essential for professionals to keep abreast of the latest innovations and their potential in order to maximise the benefits for their patients.

Continuing education and technology watch for nurses.

The world of healthcare is constantly changing. Technological advances, new medical research and societal changes are transforming the way care is delivered. Faced with this dynamic, nurses in follow-up and rehabilitation care (FCRD) need to continue their training and adopt a technology watch posture to remain at the cutting edge of their profession. Let's look at this subject in more detail.

Continuing education :
Continuing education is the cornerstone of every nurse's professional development. It ensures not only that knowledge is kept up to date, but also that new skills are acquired to meet the current demands of the profession.

- **Specialised training:** Depending on the needs of the FCRDR department or professional aspirations, nurses can choose specific training courses, for example in pain management, palliative care or the management of particular pathologies.
- **Practical workshops:** These workshops, often organised by medical institutions or specialist companies, provide an opportunity to learn and master the use of new equipment or techniques.
- **Seminars and conferences:** These provide an opportunity to keep abreast of current trends, hear from experts in the field and share experiences with other professionals.
- **Soft skills training:** These skills, such as communication, stress management and leadership, are essential for nurses who work in teams and with a variety of patients.

Technology watch :
Technology watch is the art of monitoring, analysing and taking advantage of technological innovations likely to have an impact on the healthcare sector.

- **Subscription to professional journals:** These journals are often the first to present articles on new technologies, methods or studies in the nursing field.
- **Participation in medical fairs and exhibitions:** These events showcase the latest innovations, allowing nurses to see, touch and sometimes try out new tools.
- **Professional networks:** Joining professional associations or groups on social media allows you to

discuss the latest trends with your peers and get recommendations.

- **Online training:** Many platforms offer courses on the latest technological advances in healthcare, which can be accessed at any time.
- **Partnerships with suppliers:** Some suppliers offer training courses to support the adoption of new technologies in care establishments.

It is crucial for nurses working in the CRH to take a proactive approach to continuing education and technology monitoring. This commitment not only guarantees optimum patient care, but also strengthens the nurse's professional position in a constantly changing medical environment.

Chapter 8:
ETHICAL AND LEGAL ASPECTS

Patients' rights in FCRD.

In a Continuing Care and Rehabilitation (CCR) establishment, as in any other medical setting, patients' rights are paramount. They ensure that each individual is treated with dignity and respect, and that they receive care appropriate to their condition. Let's take a closer look at these fundamental rights in the context of FCRD.

1. Right to information :
Every patient has the right to be informed about his or her condition, the treatment offered, its benefits, risks and alternatives. This information, delivered in a clear and appropriate manner, enables patients to play an active part in making decisions about their treatment.

2. Free and informed consent :
No medical procedure may be carried out without the patient's consent. Consent must be free, informed and given explicitly, except in an emergency where the patient is unable to express his or her wishes.

3. Privacy and confidentiality :
All information relating to the patient must remain confidential. FCRDR staff must respect this confidentiality, as well as the patient's right to privacy during treatment.

4. Quality of care and safety :
Every FCRD patient has the right to receive high-quality care in a safe environment. This includes complying with medical protocols, using appropriate equipment and ensuring a clean and safe environment.

5. Right to refuse or withdraw treatment :
Patients may refuse treatment or request that it be stopped at any time, even if this may have consequences for their

health. They must be informed of the repercussions of such a decision.

6. Access to medical records :
All patients have the right to access their medical records. This enables them to understand their care pathway, consult medical reports and play an active role in their care.

7. The right to pain relief :
Recognising and treating pain is fundamental. Patients have the right to have their pain assessed, taken into account and treated appropriately.

8. The right to be accompanied and supported :
In FCRD, given the prolonged and complex nature of care, the support of relatives is essential. Patients therefore have the right to be accompanied by their loved ones, while respecting the organisation of their care.

9. Expression of complaints and claims :
If patients feel that their rights have not been respected or that they are dissatisfied with the care they have received, they have the right to express their complaints and demands to the establishment, which is obliged to deal with them.

10. Respect for the end of life :
In the event of a serious, progressive and incurable illness, every patient has specific rights relating to the end of life, particularly with regard to advance directives and deep sedation.

Awareness of and respect for these rights by all those involved, including nurses, are essential to guarantee humane, ethical and high-quality care in the CRH. It is the duty of every professional to be informed and to ensure that these rights are always put forward in their daily practice.

Ethical considerations on rehabilitation and the end of life.

Rehabilitation, like the end of life, refers to sensitive periods in human existence when individuals are faced with profound challenges, choices and questions. Follow-up and rehabilitation care (FCRD) has the mission of supporting patients at these crucial moments, but they also generate important ethical reflections.

Rehabilitation: between hope and reality
- **Freedom of choice vs. optimal well-being:** How can we balance the patient's wishes (who may wish to abandon rehabilitation) with the medical need to continue rehabilitation in order to guarantee long-term well-being?
- **Dignity and autonomy:** Every patient wants to regain their autonomy, but how far should rehabilitation go to preserve this dignity?
- **Technology and humanity:** While technology offers increasing possibilities for rehabilitation, how can we ensure that the human dimension remains at the heart of the process?

The end of life: a major ethical challenge
- **Quality of life vs. prolongation of life:** When medicine can prolong life, but not necessarily its quality, what decision should be taken? And who should make it: the patient, the family, the carers?
- **Advance directives:** These are designed to respect patients' wishes regarding the end of their lives. However, how should they be interpreted when they seem to run counter to what is medically possible or optimal?
- **Emotional support:** How can you provide appropriate emotional support to patients and their

families, while preserving your own mental health as a healthcare professional?

- **The decision to stop treatment :** When is it ethical to decide to stop treatment? What role does the opinion of the patient, the family and the doctors play?

At the heart of these ethical considerations are universal values such as dignity, respect, autonomy and benevolence. Because of the care, rehabilitation and support they provide, FCRD are faced with these dilemmas on a daily basis. It is essential for healthcare professionals to take the time to reflect, train and discuss these ethical challenges with wisdom, compassion and integrity. The key lies in listening carefully and respectfully to the patient, and communicating transparently with all those involved.

Importance of documentation and confidentiality.

Documentation and confidentiality are two essential pillars in the medical field, and more particularly in the field of Follow-up and Rehabilitation Care (FCRD). They form the basis on which the relationship of trust between the patient and the medical team is built. Let's explore this duality in depth.

Documentation: at the heart of care

- **Traceability of care:** Documentation ensures complete traceability of all care and interventions carried out. This ensures continuity of care, especially in a multidisciplinary environment such as an FCRD where several professionals are involved.
- **Communication between professionals:** Rigorous documentation facilitates the sharing of information between the different members of the care team. It

provides an overview of the patient's situation, guaranteeing harmonised care.
- **Monitoring and evaluation:** Documentation is used to assess the patient's progress, adjust care plans accordingly and measure the effectiveness of interventions.
- **Legal liability: In the** event of a dispute, documentation serves as proof of the care provided and the decisions taken.

Confidentiality: a promise of integrity
- **Respect for patients' rights:** Every patient has the right to privacy. Confidentiality guarantees that personal and medical information will not be disclosed without the patient's consent.
- **Creating a space of trust:** Knowing that their information is treated confidentially encourages patients to be more open and honest about their condition, making it easier for them to receive care.
- **Professional ethics:** Confidentiality is at the heart of medical ethics. It defines the FCRD as a secure environment where respect for the patient is paramount.
- **Protection against abuse:** In our digital age, confidentiality also provides protection against potential abuse, such as identity theft or the exploitation of data for unauthorised purposes.

Documentation and confidentiality are therefore intimately linked. Accurate and complete documentation is useless if it is not treated with the strictest confidentiality. Conversely, respect for confidentiality is compromised if documentation is not rigorously maintained. Healthcare professionals, and in particular nurses in CRHs, have a major role to play in ensuring that these two elements are always respected, thereby guaranteeing optimal and ethical care for patients.

Chapter 9:
SPECIAL FEATURES POPULATIONS IN FCRD

Children in the FCRD : particularities and challenges.

Children in follow-up and rehabilitation care are a special group, with specific needs and challenges. Whether dedicated exclusively to children or as part of a wider structure, paediatric FCRD facilities are faced with a series of particularities and challenges specific to this population.

The particularities of children in FCRD
- **Changing physiology:** Children's bodies are constantly growing and developing. This means that their rehabilitation must take account of these physiological changes if it is to be effective.
- **Specific pathologies:** Certain disorders or illnesses are unique to paediatrics, and therefore require specific expertise to ensure they are treated appropriately.
- **Psychological impact:** Children are still developing cognitively and emotionally. Trauma or illness can have a profound impact on their psychological well-being, their self-image and their relationship with the world.
- **The role of the family:** For children, the family plays a key role in the rehabilitation process. Their involvement, support and training are essential.

Challenges specific to paediatric FCRD
- **Appropriate communication:** You need to be able to communicate with children at their level, using clear,

reassuring language. Therapeutic education must be adapted to their age and understanding.

- **Active participation by the child:** Involving the child in the rehabilitation process is a challenge, but it is also the key to its success. Therapeutic games and the playfulness of care can help to make this process more attractive.
- **Emotional support:** Children may not fully understand what is happening to them, or may be frightened. Providing appropriate emotional support, sometimes via professionals such as specialist psychologists, is crucial.
- **Coordination with the education system:** Alongside care, it is often necessary to coordinate rehabilitation with the child's schooling, whether to maintain academic standards or to prepare for a return to school.
- **Parent training:** Parents or guardians often need to be trained to take an active part in their child's care, particularly in the CRH setting where rehabilitation often continues at home.

The approach taken in paediatric FCRD must therefore be comprehensive, taking into account all the child's specific needs, both physical and psychological. It requires close collaboration between the various healthcare professionals, the child himself and his family, to ensure optimal care and a return to a normal life.

Geriatric FCRD : meeting needs the elderly.

Geriatric follow-up and rehabilitation care (FCRD) focuses on the care of the elderly, a population with distinct needs and issues. The challenges of geriatrics are numerous and require a holistic, tailored approach.

Particularities of elderly patients in FCRD
- **Polypathology:** Elderly people often have several simultaneous pathologies, requiring complex medical care and careful coordination between various specialists.
- **Physical vulnerability:** With age, the body loses its robustness. The bones are more fragile, the skin thinner, and the immune system is often weakened, making rehabilitation more delicate.
- **Cognitive aspects:** Cognitive disorders, such as dementia or Alzheimer's disease, can be common and require a specific approach during rehabilitation.
- **Psychosocial:** Loneliness, depression or feelings of dependence can affect the patient's state of mind and motivation, thus influencing the rehabilitation process.

Challenges and responses in geriatric FCRD
- **Individualised care:** Every senior is unique. Care must be tailored not only to the individual's pathology, but also to his or her life history, habits and wishes.
- **Interdisciplinarity:** The approach must be multidisciplinary, involving doctors, nurses, physiotherapists, occupational therapists, psychologists and other specialists to meet the patient's various needs.
- **The environment:** Creating a safe, reassuring and stimulating environment is essential. The adaptation of the physical environment and the presence of staff trained in geriatrics are key elements.
- **Active patient participation:** Despite their age, senior citizens need to play an active role in their rehabilitation. This may mean overcoming reluctance, fear or prejudice.
- **Family support:** Family and friends play an important role in the rehabilitation process. They can be a source of emotional support, but they also need to be trained to support the patient on a day-to-day basis.

- **Transition to home:** Returning home is often the goal in geriatric CRH. The aim is to prepare for this return, adapt the home if necessary and ensure that the patient and his family have the necessary tools and skills.

The FCRD gériatriques are therefore an appropriate response to the complex needs of the elderly. They offer comprehensive, person-centred care, with the aim of improving quality of life, maintaining or restoring independence, and preventing age-related complications. In this context, the human dimension of care, listening and caring are essential if we are to respond effectively to the challenges of modern geriatrics.

Rehabilitation of patients neurodegenerative diseases or trauma.

The rehabilitation of patients suffering from neurodegenerative diseases or trauma is a major medical and human challenge. The aim is to restore, maintain or optimise the level of autonomy and quality of life of these patients, despite the serious physical and cognitive consequences associated with their condition.

Neurodegenerative diseases: a battle against time
Neurodegenerative diseases, such as Alzheimer's, Parkinson's and multiple sclerosis, are characterised by the progressive deterioration of neurons. They affect mobility, cognitive ability, speech and many other vital functions.
- **Motor rehabilitation:** Specific exercises, often carried out by physiotherapists, aim to slow the progression of motor disorders, improve balance and reduce the risk of falls.
- **Cognitive stimulation:** Cognitive stimulation workshops, run in collaboration with

neuropsychologists, aim to preserve the patient's mental capacity for as long as possible.
- **Psychological support:** Faced with the progressive loss of their abilities, many patients feel anxious, depressed or frustrated. Psychological support is often necessary.

Cerebral trauma: the challenge of reconstruction
Trauma, whether caused by a stroke, head injury or tumour, can lead to a variety of after-effects.
- **Intensive therapy:** Immediately after a trauma, intensive care is often necessary to stabilise the patient's condition and prevent possible complications.
- **Motor rehabilitation:** Depending on the area of the brain affected, patients may need rehabilitation to regain their motor skills.
- **Rehabilitation of cognitive functions:** Cerebral trauma can have an impact on memory, attention, language, etc. Specific therapies are put in place to help patients recover or compensate for these functions.
- **Emotional support: The** psychological consequences of a brain injury are profound. Patients often have to let go of certain abilities and relearn to live with their new limitations.

In both cases, follow-up and rehabilitation care (FCRD) is fundamental. It offers a holistic and individualised approach, tailored to the specific needs of each patient. Collaboration between different healthcare professionals (doctors, nurses, physiotherapists, occupational therapists, neuropsychologists, etc.) is essential to provide comprehensive care. Rehabilitation is a complex journey, made up of progress, plateaus and sometimes regressions, but with the constant objective of the patient's well-being and autonomy.

Chapter 10:
PREVENTION
AND THERAPEUTIC EDUCATION

The importance of preventing complications.

Preventing complications in follow-up and rehabilitation care is of paramount importance. In this context of rehabilitation, patients are often in a convalescence phase or in a vulnerable situation due to a chronic illness or traumatic event. The occurrence of complications can seriously compromise the recovery process, lengthening the length of stay, reducing quality of life and, in some cases, threatening the prognosis.

Prevention focuses on several key areas:

1. Continuous monitoring :
The medical and care teams carry out rigorous monitoring to rapidly detect any signs of deterioration in the patient's condition. This may involve regular check-ups, taking vital signs and appropriate tests.

2. Hygiene and infection prevention :
Hospital-acquired infections are a major concern in hospitals. Strict compliance with hygiene protocols, staff training and patient and family education are essential to limit the risks.

3. Pressure sore prevention :
Patients who are bedridden or have reduced mobility are at risk of developing pressure sores. Particular attention is paid to changing position, using suitable mattresses and skin care.

4. Appropriate nutrition :
A balanced diet tailored to the patient's needs is essential to boost the immune system, promote recovery and prevent complications such as malnutrition.

5. Early mobilisation :
Depending on the situation, it may be beneficial to mobilise the patient as early as possible to prevent muscular or joint complications and stimulate blood circulation.

6. Falls prevention :
Falls can lead to fractures and other injuries. It is therefore crucial to assess the risk, adapt the environment and educate the patient and family.

7. Therapeutic education :
Informing patients about their illness, treatment and the precautions to be taken allows them to be actively involved in their recovery and prevents certain complications.

8. Care coordination :
Multidisciplinarity is a major strength of FCRD. Communication between the various professionals (doctors, nurses, physiotherapists, occupational therapists, etc.) guarantees comprehensive and appropriate care.

In addition to physiological complications, it is also important to anticipate and prevent psychological complications such as feelings of isolation, depression and anxiety. Care in the FCRD must be comprehensive, taking into account both the physical and psychological needs of the patient.

Preventing complications in CRH is not only a medical necessity, but also an ethical approach aimed at offering patients the best possible quality of care, respect for their dignity and the best possible prognosis for recovery.

Therapeutic patient education : a key role for nurses.

Therapeutic patient education (TPE) is a cornerstone of modern medical care. Its aim is to empower patients to take charge of their own health, giving them the tools they need to understand their illness and treatment, adapt their behaviour and cope with difficult situations. Nurses play a central role in this process.

The nurse: an educator who listens
Nurses are often the health professional closest to the patient. They are present on a daily basis, providing care, listening and responding to concerns. This proximity makes them an ideal educator for establishing a climate of trust with patients.

Passing on appropriate knowledge
Nurses provide clear, accessible information about the disease, treatments and their side-effects, as well as the possible evolution of the pathology. In doing so, they help patients to deconstruct preconceived ideas and build a solid body of knowledge tailored to their specific situation.
Developing skills
As well as imparting knowledge, ETP aims to develop practical skills. For example, nurses can teach patients how to take their medication correctly, recognise and manage symptoms, and adapt their diet or physical activity.
Encouraging patient autonomy
The ultimate aim of TVE is to enable patients to manage their illness independently. Thanks to the nurse's interventions, patients learn to make informed decisions about their health, anticipate and manage crises, and adapt to changes in their condition.

Teamwork

Although nurses play a central role in TVE, they never work alone. They work closely with doctors, physiotherapists, occupational therapists, psychologists and other professionals to provide coherent, comprehensive education.

Adapting to each patient

Each patient is unique, with his or her own history, culture, beliefs, fears and hopes. Nurses must be empathetic, good listeners and flexible enough to adapt their approach and methods to each individual.

A long-term commitment

Therapeutic education is not a one-off event, but an ongoing process. Patients' needs and questions evolve over time, as do medical and scientific advances. The nurse's regular presence with the patient ensures that TVE is updated and reinforced throughout the patient's care.

Nurses are much more than just care providers. They are the patient's true partner, guiding them in understanding and managing their illness. Therapeutic education, with its informative, formative and relational dimensions, magnifies the role of the nurse as an essential player in the overall care of the patient.

Teaching techniques and methods adapted to the patient.

The effectiveness of therapeutic education depends to a large extent on the healthcare professional's ability to adapt his or her teaching methods and techniques to each individual patient. The target audience in a medical context is often heterogeneous, with varying levels of education, cultural backgrounds, ages and cognitive abilities. Here are a few techniques and methods that can be used for tailored therapeutic education:

1. Initial needs and skills assessment :
Before any teaching begins, it is essential to assess the patient's prior knowledge, beliefs, skills and needs. This enables the teaching to be adapted to each individual.
2. Use of simple, clear language :
Avoid medical jargon and explain concepts in a way that everyone can understand.

3. Active learning methods :
Involve the patient in the learning process. This can be done through discussions, role-playing, role-playing, practical workshops, etc.

4. Visual aids :
Diagrams, infographics, videos and demonstrations can help to make information more tangible, especially for those who learn best visually.

5. Step-by-step teaching :
Break the information down into easily digestible segments or stages. This makes it easier to assimilate and allows you to build up your skills gradually.

6. Constructive feedback :
Give patients regular feedback on their skills and progress. This builds confidence and motivates further learning.

7. Repetition and reinforcement :
Regularly revisit key information and skills to ensure that they are firmly memorised.

8. Peer learning :
Encourage patients to share their experiences and advice. They can often provide unique support and insight.

9. Use of technology :
Online platforms, mobile applications and educational games can be invaluable tools for complementing and reinforcing teaching.

10. Cultural adaptation :
Ensure that teaching is adapted to patients' beliefs, values and cultural backgrounds. This may require specific training or collaboration with cultural mediators.

11. Relaxation and concentration methods :
Techniques such as meditation, deep breathing or progressive muscle relaxation can help some patients to concentrate and integrate information.

12. Continuous assessment :
Set up regular assessments to measure progress, identify areas for improvement and adjust teaching techniques accordingly.

Patient-centred teaching is as much an art as a science. It requires listening, patience, flexibility and a constant willingness to innovate to meet the unique needs of each individual. The aim is always to empower patients to understand, manage and make informed decisions about their health.

Chapter 11:
MENTAL HEALTH IN THE FCRD

Recognising and managing problems
mental health
in rehabilitation patients.

Rehabilitation is a complex process that is not limited to the physical dimension of the patient. Mental health plays a crucial role in the recovery process. Rehabilitation patients can face considerable emotional and psychological challenges, which it is essential to recognise and manage in order to optimise their chances of success.

Recognition of mental health problems :
- **Depressive symptoms:** These can include sadness, loss of interest in activities, feelings of uselessness, disturbed sleep or appetite, and even suicidal thoughts.
- **Anxiety:** Excessive worry, palpitations, trembling, excessive sweating or avoidance of certain situations are common signs.
- **Post-traumatic stress disorder (PTSD):** Patients who have suffered trauma, either at the onset of their need for rehabilitation or previously, may experience flashbacks, nightmares or hypervigilance.
- **Cognitive impairment:** Problems with memory, concentration or decision-making can occur, often as a result of brain trauma or other neurological conditions.
- **Denial or minimisation:** Some patients may refuse to accept the reality of their condition or minimise its impact.

Management of mental health problems :
- **Regular assessment:** Using standardised assessment tools and checklists can help to quickly identify signs and symptoms of psychological distress.
- **Individual therapy:** Providing a safe space for patients to talk about their feelings and concerns with a trained professional.
- **Support groups:** Support groups allow patients to share their experiences, learn from others and feel less isolated.
- **Pharmacological interventions:** Some patients may benefit from medication to treat specific disorders such as depression or anxiety.
- **Relaxation and stress management techniques:** meditation, deep breathing, biofeedback and music therapy can all be useful tools.
- **Education:** Informing patients about the links between physical and mental health, and the importance of looking after their emotional well-being.
- **Collaboration:** Working closely with psychiatrists, psychologists, social workers and other mental health professionals to ensure comprehensive care.
- **Individualised care plans:** Every patient is unique. Intervention plans must be adapted to the specific needs, preferences and circumstances of each individual.
- **Encourage physical activity:** Exercise has been shown to improve mood and reduce anxiety.
- **Access to external resources:** Provide information on community resources, helplines or emergency services in case of need.

Recognising and managing mental health problems in rehabilitation patients is essential for their overall well-being. A holistic approach, which takes into account both the physical and psychological dimensions, is the key to successful recovery.

Working with professionals mental health.

Collaboration with mental health professionals is a fundamental dimension of rehabilitation care. A patient's road to recovery is not limited to physical healing; it also encompasses emotional and psychological well-being, which are just as crucial to a return to a full and satisfying life.

In the context of Continuing Care and Rehabilitation (CCR), this collaboration becomes essential. Patients can be faced with considerable emotional challenges, whether it be pain, adapting to a new physical reality, or dealing with a recent trauma. Mental health professionals, such as psychiatrists, psychologists, psychotherapists and social workers, bring their specific expertise to bear in navigating these sometimes tumultuous waters.

But for this collaboration to be truly effective, it is vital to adopt an integrated approach. Teams need to communicate openly and regularly, exchanging key information about the patient's condition, progress made and obstacles encountered. Interdisciplinary brainstorming sessions can be particularly fruitful, blending perspectives to develop individualised, holistic intervention plans.

It is also essential to create an environment where patients feel comfortable talking about their emotional and psychological concerns, knowing that they are taken seriously and considered an integral part of their recovery journey. The approach must be one of empathy, respect and understanding.

Finally, this collaboration between healthcare professionals and mental health professionals is not limited to the period of hospitalisation or rehabilitation. For many patients, mental health support is an ongoing process, requiring regular consultations long after their discharge from the FCRD. Ensuring a smooth transition between the FCRD and outpatient mental health services is crucial to ensuring continuity of care.

In an ideal world, the line between physical and mental health would be blurred, with each dimension seen as an inseparable facet of overall wellbeing. Collaboration between health and mental health professionals is not only beneficial; it is essential if patients are to be offered the best possible recovery pathway.

Self-care strategies for nurses dealing with stress and intense emotions.

Working in Continuing Care and Rehabilitation (CCR) can be a particularly emotionally intense experience for nurses. Faced with the daily challenges, pain and hopes of patients, as well as the pressures inherent in the medical environment, the importance of self-care for nurses cannot be underestimated. Adopting self-care strategies not only helps to preserve mental health, but also to provide the best possible care for patients.

Self-care begins with recognition. It is vital for nurses to recognise and accept that stress and intense emotions are an integral part of their work. This acceptance is the first step in actively managing these pressures.

Emotional regulation is an essential skill. It involves learning to identify your emotions, understand them and express them appropriately. Techniques such as deep breathing, meditation or even taking a break during the day can help to refocus the mind.

Establishing clear boundaries between professional and personal life is crucial. While dedication to one's profession is laudable, it is essential to take time for oneself, to disconnect, recharge and engage in activities that provide pleasure and relaxation.

Peer supervision and discussion provide a space for sharing experiences, frustrations and successes. Talking to colleagues who understand the specific challenges of the profession can offer invaluable support.

Regular training in stress management and emotional skills can provide valuable tools for coping with the challenges of the job. Such training can take the form of seminars, workshops or even one-to-one sessions with a mental health professional.

Regular physical activity is an excellent way to relieve stress. Whether it's yoga, running, dancing or any other form of exercise, movement can help relieve accumulated stress and leave you feeling revitalised.

Diet and sleep are two pillars of overall health. A balanced diet and quality sleep are essential for coping with daily stress and ensuring optimum performance at work.

Striking a balance between professional and personal life is also fundamental. It's important to remember that, just as patients need care, carers also need time for themselves, time with their families, leisure time or simply rest.

Finally, **acceptance**. It's important to remember that nobody is perfect. Recognising your limits, accepting that you can't control everything and seeking help when you need it are signs of strength, not weakness.

The mental and emotional health of nurses is essential to the quality of the care they provide. Adopting self-care strategies is not a luxury, but a necessity for these dedicated professionals.

Chapter 12:
THE CULTURAL DIMENSION IN THE FCRD

Understanding and respecting the cultural diversity of patients.

In today's increasingly globalised world, nurses in the Continuing Care and Rehabilitation (CCR) sector are often called upon to care for patients from a variety of cultural backgrounds. Understanding and respecting this cultural diversity is not only a question of ethics, but also a key element in providing high-quality, personalised care.

Cultural diversity is not just about nationality or language. It also encompasses religious beliefs, traditions, family values, eating habits, perceptions of health and illness, and many other aspects. These elements can influence the way a patient perceives their illness, their recovery, their expectations of care, and even the way they communicate with healthcare professionals.

The importance of intercultural training is paramount. Nurses should be encouraged and trained to understand different cultures, not to categorise them, but to offer adapted and individualised care. Such training can help to deconstruct stereotypes and prevent misunderstandings.

Communication is key. It is crucial to listen actively to patients, ask open questions and encourage dialogue. If language barriers are an obstacle, consider using medical interpreters to ensure clear communication.

Cultural sensitivity involves being aware of one's own prejudices and attitudes, and striving to understand the patient's point of view. For example, some patients may have spiritual or traditional beliefs about the causes of illness or methods of healing, and it is crucial to approach these with respect and an open mind.

Taking cultural diversity into account in the care plan is essential. This may mean adjusting diets to suit cultural preferences, understanding religious or spiritual rituals around healing, or adapting therapeutic education methods to make them culturally relevant.

Collaboration with the family and the community can enrich the care experience. In many cultures, the family plays a central role in the healing process, and integrating this dynamic can improve adherence to treatment and the patient's well-being.

Respect and dignity are universal. Whatever a patient's culture, treating them with respect and dignity is fundamental. This means respecting confidentiality, asking permission before any intervention, and always acting with empathy.

At the end of the day, embracing cultural diversity is about humanity and inclusion. It recognises that each patient is unique, with his or her own history, beliefs and values. In the field of FCRD, where rehabilitation is a complex and deeply personal journey, this recognition is even more crucial. It is by embracing cultural diversity that nurses can offer truly holistic, patient-centred care.

Techniques intercultural communication.

Intercultural communication techniques are essential for nurses and other healthcare professionals. They enable them to understand and respond effectively to the needs of patients from different cultural backgrounds. Adopting effective intercultural communication means ensuring patient-centred care, while strengthening the therapeutic bond.

1. Self-awareness: Before we can understand others, it is crucial to become aware of our own biases, prejudices and values. Reflecting on our own culture and how it influences our perception of others is the first step towards effective intercultural communication.

2. Active listening: Active listening means paying full attention to what the other person is saying, without interruption. It helps to identify the patient's specific needs and to recognise any misunderstandings.

3. Patience: Communicating with patients from different cultures can take longer, especially if there is a language barrier. It is important to be patient and not to rush the conversation.

4. The use of interpreters : In situations where language is a barrier, the use of a trained medical interpreter is essential. The interpreter not only translates words, but also cultural nuances.

5. Ask open-ended questions: These questions encourage dialogue and allow you to obtain more detailed information. They can also help to clarify points of ambiguity.

6. Avoid medical jargon: It is preferable to use simple, clear language, avoiding as far as possible technical jargon that may not be understood.

7. Observe non-verbal language: Non-verbal communication, such as gestures, facial expressions and posture, plays a key role in intercultural understanding. Certain expressions or gestures can have different meanings in different cultures.

8. Respect cultural beliefs and practices: This may concern a variety of aspects, such as food preferences, religious practices or beliefs about health and illness.

9. Provide visual aids : Pictures, diagrams and other visual aids can make it easier to understand, especially when there is a language barrier.

10. Information and training: Taking part in training courses on intercultural communication and keeping abreast of the cultures present in the community served can greatly improve interactions with patients.

11. Establish trust: This is fundamental to successful communication. Listening with respect, showing empathy and guaranteeing confidentiality are all ways of establishing and maintaining this trust.

Ultimately, intercultural communication requires a patient-centred approach based on respect, empathy and a willingness to understand. It is by embracing these techniques and integrating them into their daily practice that nurses and other healthcare professionals can ensure quality care for all their patients, whatever their cultural background.

Ethics and cultural sensitivity in care.

Ethics and cultural sensitivity are fundamental pillars of nursing practice. Integrating them into care ensures that every patient receives respectful, understanding and individualised care. In a context of globalisation and increasingly diverse populations, the ability to adapt clinical practice to patients' cultural needs is essential.

Ethics in care :
Ethics refer to the moral principles that guide our conduct. In the medical world, it aims to guarantee the well-being and respect of patients.
- **Autonomy:** Every patient has the right to make decisions about his or her own care, after having been appropriately informed. This means respecting individual choices and values.
- **Beneficence:** The aim of care is to provide a benefit to the patient, while minimising potential risks and harm.

- **Non-maleficence:** "Do no harm" is a cardinal principle. Healthcare professionals must strive to avoid unnecessary or potentially harmful interventions.
- **Justice:** Care must be administered equitably, guaranteeing access to treatment and the necessary resources for all.

Cultural sensitivity in care :
Cultural sensitivity refers to the ability to recognise and respect cultural differences, and to integrate them into care.
- **Recognition:** Understanding that each individual is the product of their own cultural context, with their own beliefs, values and practices.
- **Curiosity:** Finding out more about patients' traditions, customs and beliefs so that we can better meet their needs.
- **Respect:** Approaching each patient without judgement, valuing their experience and culture.
- **Adaptability:** Adjusting care to the patient's cultural needs, whether in terms of dietary preferences, religious practices or health beliefs.
- **Ongoing training:** Regularly take part in cultural sensitivity training courses to stay informed and competent.

The intersection of ethics and cultural sensitivity :
When ethics meet culture, dilemmas can arise. For example, how do you manage a situation where a patient's cultural beliefs conflict with medical recommendations? In these situations, communication is key. It is essential to establish an open dialogue with the patient and their family, seeking to understand their perspectives while sharing the necessary medical information. The aim is to arrive at a care plan that respects both ethical principles and cultural values.

Combining ethics and cultural sensitivity means engaging in holistic, patient-centred nursing practice. This is an ongoing process, requiring reflection, training and adaptation, but it is also the key to providing the best possible quality of care for all patients.

Chapter 13:
INNOVATIONS AND RESEARCH IN FCRD

The latest advances in rehabilitation.

Rehabilitation has seen major advances in recent years, both in therapeutic approaches and in the technologies used. The aim of these innovations is to improve patients' quality of life and help them regain their independence as fully as possible.

1. Virtual and augmented reality technologies :
Virtual reality (VR) and augmented reality (AR) are increasingly used in rehabilitation, particularly to treat motor or cognitive disorders. Thanks to interactive simulations, patients can practise certain tasks or exercises in a controlled, adaptable environment.

2. Telerehabilitation :
Telemedicine has paved the way for telerehabilitation, enabling patients to benefit from rehabilitation sessions at a distance, using online platforms. This is particularly useful for those who live far from rehabilitation centres or who have difficulty travelling.

3. Exoskeletons and rehabilitation robots :
These technological devices help patients to regain their motor skills, particularly after an accident or surgery. They enable more precise rehabilitation, tailored to each patient, and can speed up the recovery process.

4. Neuroplasticity and brain stimulation :
A growing understanding of neuroplasticity - the brain's ability to reorganise itself and create new neuronal connections - has led to the development of non-invasive brain stimulation techniques. These methods, such as transcranial magnetic stimulation, can help to improve cognitive and motor functions.

5. Biofeedback :

This technique uses electronic equipment to inform the patient in real time about certain physiological functions, enabling them to modulate them. It is particularly useful for pain management, perineal rehabilitation and the treatment of certain neurological disorders.

6. New-generation prostheses and implants :

Thanks to technological advances, prostheses are becoming increasingly sophisticated, with thought-controlled bionic prostheses and implants that restore certain sensations.

7. Integrative therapeutic approaches :

Alternative therapies, such as acupuncture, meditation or art therapy, are gaining in popularity as part of rehabilitation programmes, as they offer complementary ways of dealing with the physical, mental and emotional aspects of rehabilitation.

8. Patient-centred training :

This is an approach in which the patient is actively involved in making decisions about their own treatment. This can increase commitment and improve rehabilitation outcomes.

9. Advanced imaging techniques :

Tools such as functional MRI and positron emission tomography provide a better understanding of how the brain works and enable rehabilitation interventions to be adapted.

These advances, combined with a better understanding of the body's recovery mechanisms, mean that rehabilitation care can be offered that is ever more personalised and effective. They represent immense hope for many patients who aspire to return to a normal life after illness, injury or surgery.

Implications of new discoveries for nursing practice.

New discoveries and advances in the field of rehabilitation have significant implications for nursing practice, transforming the way care is delivered and how nurses interact with their patients and colleagues. Here are some of the key implications of these discoveries for nursing practice:

1. The need for continuing education :
With the emergence of new technologies and techniques, nurses need to constantly update their skills and knowledge. This means regularly attending specialist training courses, workshops and seminars.

2. Holistic approach to care :
New rehabilitation methods recognise the importance of treating the patient as a whole, physically, psychologically and socially. Nurses must therefore develop a thorough understanding of these aspects in order to provide truly patient-centred care.

3. Enhanced collaboration :
Rehabilitation care is becoming increasingly interdisciplinary. Nurses work closely with other health professionals, such as physiotherapists, occupational therapists, psychologists and even biomedical engineers. Effective communication and mutual understanding are essential.

4. Technology for care :
Nurses need to familiarise themselves with technological tools, whether for telerehabilitation, the use of biofeedback devices or the interpretation of advanced imaging results. Mastery of these technologies is essential for optimal care.

5. Patient education and awareness :

With the availability of innovative tools and techniques, nurses play a crucial role in patient education, helping patients to understand and navigate this changing medical landscape.

6. Ethics and confidentiality :

The increasing use of technology also raises ethical issues, particularly in terms of data confidentiality and access to information. Nurses need to be aware of the regulations in force and ensure that professional ethics are respected.

7. Mental health :

Integrating psychological aspects into rehabilitation care means paying greater attention to patients' mental health. Nurses must be trained to recognise and address these issues, working with specialists where necessary.

8. Personalised care :

With a better understanding of individual recovery mechanisms and the availability of advanced technologies, care can be more personalised. Nurses must therefore be able to adapt their approach to the specific needs of each patient.

9. Prevention and education :

With their knowledge of risk factors and prevention methods, nurses have a key role to play in educating patients about preventive measures, thereby helping to reduce the need for subsequent interventions.

As the world of rehabilitation continues to evolve, nurses remain at the heart of care, constantly adapting their skills and adopting a patient-centred approach to ensure the best possible care.

How to stay up to date
in a rapidly evolving field.

Staying up to date in an ever-changing field like healthcare is crucial to providing optimal care and maintaining professional relevance. Here are some strategies to help professionals, especially nurses, navigate a rapidly changing medical landscape:

1. Continuing education :
Sign up regularly for training courses, workshops and seminars specialising in your field. Numerous institutions and professional associations offer training adapted to the latest advances.

2. Subscriptions to professional journals :
Medical and nursing journals are excellent resources for the latest research and recommendations. Subscribe to a few relevant journals and take the time to read them regularly.

3. Taking part in conferences and congresses:
These events often bring together renowned experts to share their research and knowledge. As well as acquiring new information, you'll be able to network with other professionals.

4. Get involved in professional groups:
Join professional associations or think tanks. These groups often offer resources, training and discussion forums for sharing experience and knowledge.

5. Use :
Online platforms, webinars and MOOCs (Massive Open Online Courses) can offer distance learning opportunities. There are many applications and educational platforms dedicated to healthcare professionals.

6. Keep abreast of technological developments:
Keep an eye on technological innovations that may have an impact on your field. This could include new equipment, software or processing techniques.

7. Reciprocal teaching :
Teaching others or mentoring students can help you strengthen your own knowledge. The act of teaching requires a deep understanding, which means you need to stay informed.

8. Talk to your colleagues:
Regular exchanges with your peers can expose you to different perspectives and experiences. Organise or take part in discussion groups or team meetings to share knowledge.

9. Get involved in research :
If possible, get involved in research projects or work with researchers. This will keep you at the cutting edge of advances in your field.

10. Adopt a lifelong learner attitude:
Recognising that learning never stops is crucial. Be open to change, adapt and be proactive in your quest for knowledge.

In an ever-changing medical environment, the key is to adopt a proactive stance, regularly engaging in learning activities and actively seeking opportunities to improve and update your skills.

Chapter 14:
END-OF-LIFE MANAGEMENT
IN THE FCRD

Navigating difficult decisions and conversations about the end of life.

Navigating difficult decisions and broaching end-of-life conversations are among the most delicate and complex tasks facing healthcare professionals. These moments require deep sensitivity, attentive listening and a solid ethical understanding. Here's how to approach these situations with empathy and professionalism:

1. Creating a comfortable environment :
Before starting such a conversation, make sure that the environment is calm, private and free from distractions. A peaceful setting can help facilitate a calm discussion.

2. Prepare yourself emotionally:
Acknowledge your own emotions and beliefs on the subject. Being aware of your own feelings can help you approach the conversation with greater objectivity and empathy.

3. Listen before you speak :
Start by asking the patient or family how they perceive the current situation. Giving them the floor first can help set the tone of the conversation.

4. Use simple, clear language:
Avoid medical jargon and be direct yet sensitive. Make sure the patient and family understand the situation.

5. Be empathetic :
Acknowledge and validate the emotions of the patient and their family. Phrases such as "I can imagine how difficult this must be for you" or "I'm here to support you" can offer some comfort.

6. Ask open-ended questions:

Encourage the patient and family to express their concerns, wishes and feelings by asking questions such as "How do you see the next steps?" or "What is most important to you right now?".

7. Provide information on all the options :

Make sure the patient and family are well informed of all the options available, including palliative care, refusal of treatment, etc.

8. Respect the patient's choices :

Everyone has the right to make decisions about their own care. As long as the patient is able to make an informed decision, it is crucial to respect their wishes, even if you personally do not agree.

9. Provide ongoing support :

Feelings and decisions can change over time. Make sure the patient and family know that they can always come back to you to discuss or revisit the decisions they have made.

10. Take care of yourself:

Conversations about the end of life can be emotionally draining for healthcare professionals. Find ways to take care of yourself, whether by talking to a colleague, consulting a mental health professional or practising meditation and other relaxation techniques.

Navigating through these discussions requires a combination of clinical skill, compassion and listening. With the right training and an empathetic attitude, healthcare professionals can help patients and their families get through these difficult times with dignity and respect.

The importance of palliative care in CRD.

Palliative care, which focuses on pain management and symptom relief for patients in the advanced stages of an illness, is not just for end-of-life services. In fact, it plays a crucial role in follow-up and rehabilitation care (FCRD), where the main aim is to help patients regain as much autonomy as possible after acute hospitalisation or in the face of serious pathologies.

The integration of palliative care in FCRD :
- **Holistic patient care:** Palliative care offers a holistic approach, taking into account not only the patient's physical needs, but also their psychological, social and spiritual needs. This approach is in line with the objectives of FCRD, which aim to provide comprehensive care for patients in order to optimise their quality of life.
- **Pain management:** In an FCRD department, many patients suffer from chronic or complex pain. The principles of palliative care, with its expertise in pain management, are therefore essential to ensure patient comfort and promote rehabilitation.
- **Emotional support:** Palliative care places particular emphasis on psychological support. In FCRD, where patients may be confronted with major upheavals in their lives following a medical event, this psychological dimension is essential.
- **Informed decision-making:** Professionals trained in palliative care have the skills to lead in-depth discussions about the patient's wishes, hopes, fears and goals, which is essential for defining an appropriate therapeutic plan in the CRH.
- **Link with families:** Palliative care also focuses on the patient's family and loved ones, seeing them as an integral part of the care process. This approach is particularly beneficial in FCRD, where family support can play a major role in the patient's rehabilitation process.
- **Ethics and end of life:** Although not all patients in the CRH are terminally ill, some may be faced with a

rapid deterioration in their state of health. In these cases, palliative care expertise is essential in navigating complex ethical decisions and offering patients a dignified end of life that respects their wishes.

Palliative care, with its patient-centred approach and comprehensive pain and symptom management, greatly enriches the FCRD framework. Its integration ensures that every patient, whatever their needs or stage of illness, receives appropriate, humane and respectful care.

Supporting patients and their families in their final moments.

Accompanying patients and their families during their final moments is undoubtedly one of the most delicate and profound tasks in a healthcare professional's career. This period is saturated with intense emotions, questions, uncertainties and often a search for meaning. The role of the carer extends far beyond medical care to become a pillar of emotional, spiritual and human support. Here's how to approach this support with sensitivity, compassion and professionalism.

1. Transparent and empathetic communication :
Honest communication with patients and their families is crucial. Use simple, understandable language, while remaining sensitive to everyone's emotional state. Be an active listener, allowing the patient and family to express themselves, ask questions and share their feelings.

2. Pain management :
One of the most important aspects of end-of-life care is pain management and patient comfort. Make sure that the necessary medicines and interventions are available to minimise suffering.

3. Psychological support :

The end of life is a time of reflection, memories and sometimes regret. Offering psychological support, whether through active listening or a mental health professional, is essential.

4. Respect for beliefs and values :

Everyone has their own concept of death, often influenced by culture, religion or personal experience. Respect these beliefs and ensure that patients are given the opportunity, if possible, to practise their rites and rituals.

5. Privacy :

Allow the patient and their family to share intimate moments, respecting their need for tranquillity. This can include creating a quiet space, listening to music or lighting candles, depending on the patient's wishes.

6. Family inclusion :

The family plays a central role in the final moments. Guide them on how to interact with the patient, reassure them and also offer them emotional support.

7. Preparing for bereavement :

The period leading up to death can be seen as an anticipatory phase of grief for the family. Offer resources, advice and guidance to help loved ones navigate through this process.

8. A dignified departure :

All aspects of end-of-life care must aim to ensure a peaceful, comfortable and dignified death for the patient. Every gesture, every word, every decision should be guided by this principle.

Supporting patients and their families in their final moments is an immense responsibility, requiring profound humanity, sincere empathy and unconditional respect. It is at these intense moments that the role of the carer transcends mere medical practice to touch the very essence of the human condition.

Chapter 15:
TRANSITION AND DISCHARGE FROM THE FCRD

Preparing patients and their families at the exit.

Preparing patients and their families for discharge from a Continuing Care and Rehabilitation (CCR) service is a crucial stage that requires a comprehensive and individualised approach. The aim is to ensure that patients can continue their convalescence, rehabilitation or care independently or with the necessary support at home, in another establishment, or in an environment suited to their condition.

1. Assessment of the patient's level of autonomy :
Above all, it is important to assess the patient's degree of autonomy. This assessment must cover the patient's physical, mental and emotional capacities. It is on this basis that a discharge strategy will be drawn up.

2. Post-hospital planning :
Draw up a post-hospitalisation care plan in collaboration with the patient, their family and, if necessary, their GP. This plan will detail the medication, therapies required, upcoming medical appointments and any other relevant aspects of the patient's care.

3. Education and training :
Make sure that the patient and his or her family have a good understanding of home care, the use of medical equipment, how to take medicines and how to recognise the warning signs that would require urgent medical attention.

4. Coordination with external healthcare professionals :
Organise the necessary links, whether with home nurses, physiotherapists, Caregivers or any other relevant professional.

5. Home improvements :
If necessary, advise the patient and their family on what needs to be done at home to ensure the patient's safety and comfort: grab rails, access ramp, healthcare bed, etc.

6. Psychological support :
Returning home can be a source of anxiety or apprehension. Suggest resources or referrals for psychological support if necessary.

7. Setting up a monitoring system :
Clearly define how the patient's medical care will be organised. This may involve home visits, regular outpatient appointments, or a combination of both.

8. Availability and communication :
Assure patients and their families that they can contact the service if they have any questions or concerns. Leave contact details and specify the procedures.

9. Emotional preparation :
Leaving hospital is a big step. It can be both exciting and frightening for the patient and their loved ones. Take the time to discuss the emotions associated with this change and to reassure the patient about the next steps.

10. Documentation :
Provide all the necessary documents: prescriptions, medical report, recommendations for the future, etc. Make sure that the patient and his or her family understand these documents and can keep them in a safe place.

Preparing patients and their families for discharge from an FCRD is a fundamental step in ensuring a smooth transition to the next stage of their care. Careful, attentive and thorough preparation helps to avoid potential complications and ensures continuity of care under the best possible conditions.

Ensuring a smooth transition to other services or home.

Ensuring a smooth transition for a patient leaving a Continuing Care and Rehabilitation (CCR) department for another department or home is a highly responsible task. This transition stage is often a vulnerable time for the patient, who may be marked by uncertainty, anxiety or fear of leaving a secure environment. The challenge for carers is to ensure that this transition is as smooth, transparent and reassuring as possible.

1. Early preparation :
The first step to a successful transition is to prepare well in advance. Advance preparation enables the patient's needs to be identified, the necessary resources to be put in place and any potential obstacles to be anticipated.

2. Clear and continuous communication :
It is essential to establish open communication with patients and their families throughout the process. Keeping them regularly informed of upcoming stages, administrative procedures and any possible changes reassures them and establishes a climate of trust.

3. Interdisciplinary collaboration:
A successful transition often requires the involvement of several professionals: doctors, nurses, social workers, physiotherapists, etc. Effective coordination between these different players is crucial.

4. Patient training and education :
To feel safe, patients need to understand their condition, the care they must continue to receive and how to administer it. Workshops, information sessions or even demonstrations can be organised.

5. Assessment of needs at home :
If the patient returns home, it is important to assess the need for specific home adaptations, or whether home help will be required.

6. Post-transition follow-up :
Regular follow-up after the patient has been discharged ensures that everything is going well, answers any questions and adjusts the care plan if necessary.

7. Resources and referrals :
Providing the patient with a list of resources and contacts can be very useful. Whether for home services, support groups or specialist consultations, having this information at hand is reassuring.

8. Complete documentation :
On discharge, the patient must receive a complete file including medical reports, prescriptions, post-hospitalization instructions and any other relevant information.

9. Availability to respond to concerns:
Assuring the patient that they can contact the service if they need to reinforces the feeling of security. The transition does not end once the patient leaves the hospital.

Ensuring a smooth transition involves a holistic, patient-centred approach that requires preparation, communication and collaboration between all the players involved. It is an essential step in ensuring continuity of care, preserving patient well-being and optimising medical outcomes.

Post-FCRD follow-up : ensure continuity of care.

Post-rehabilitation care is an essential stage in guaranteeing continuity of care. It consolidates the progress made during the FCRD stay and helps prevent any risk of unnecessary re-hospitalisation. This phase, which is often neglected or underestimated, is an essential link in the patient's care pathway.

After a stay in an FCRD, patients may still be in a fragile state, even though they have improved. Care must therefore be planned and organised well beyond the doors of the care establishment. The transition from hospital to home or to another care facility is a real challenge, requiring seamless coordination between the various healthcare players.

Adapting to a new environment, managing care at home and resuming a professional or social activity are all stages that can be sources of stress, questions and even complications for the patient. Hence the importance of comprehensive care and rigorous monitoring.

1. Drawing up a post-FCRD care plan :
Even before the patient leaves the hospital, a care plan must be drawn up. This includes all the medical recommendations, treatments to be continued, appointments to be scheduled, as well as any adjustments that may need to be made to the home.

2. Coordination with healthcare professionals :
GPs, home care nurses, physiotherapists, pharmacists and other professionals need to work together. Information must flow smoothly between them to ensure that care is relevant and effective.

3. Psychological support :
Returning home can be a source of anxiety for patients and their families. The provision of psychological support can be beneficial in helping to overcome the emotional and psychological challenges following hospitalisation.

4. Providing resources and tools:
Tools, such as mobile applications or online platforms, can be used to monitor patients' progress, remind them of appointments or even answer their questions.

5. Follow-up visits :
These are used to regularly assess the patient's state of

health, adjust treatments if necessary and ensure that the patient understands and adheres to their care plan.

6. Therapeutic education :

This plays a fundamental role. A well-informed patient is in a better position to understand and actively participate in his or her own care, thereby optimising the chances of success of post-FCRD follow-up.

7. Anticipating complications :

Thanks to increased vigilance and effective communication with the patient, it is possible to quickly identify any signs of complications and intervene before the situation worsens.

8. Social and professional integration:

Where possible, it is essential to encourage patients to resume their social and professional activities. This contributes not only to the patient's well-being but also to his or her overall rehabilitation.

Post-FCRD follow-up is a multi-dimensional process that requires a patient-centred approach and close collaboration between all those involved. Far from being a mere formality, this phase is essential to guarantee continuity and quality of care, and thus contribute to a better prognosis for the patient.

Chapter 16:
REFLECTIONS ON THE COVID-19 PANDEMIC AND ITS IMPACT ON FCRD

The challenges posed by the pandemic.

The pandemic, which has shaken the entire world, has posed enormous challenges for the healthcare system, and in particular for Continuing Care and Rehabilitation (CCR). It has highlighted the need for unprecedented adaptability and resilience in the face of a major health crisis. While every medical sector has felt the impact of the pandemic, the FCRD sector has been faced with specific challenges that have tested both its infrastructure and its staff.

1. Overcrowding :
With the postponement of numerous surgical operations and medical treatments, FCRD departments had to adapt to a sudden and unforeseen influx of patients. Although these patients had recovered from the acute phase of their illness, they often required intensive rehabilitation, particularly after hospitalisation in an intensive care unit.

2. Increased health precautions :
Hygiene and safety protocols had to be reinforced. This meant ongoing training for staff, adaptation of premises, acquisition and management of personal protective equipment (PPE) and constant vigilance to prevent any transmission.

3. Emotional support :
The pandemic caused massive psychological distress among patients and their families. FCRD professionals, already used to dealing with emotionally intense situations, had to redouble their efforts to support patients through the trauma of illness, isolation and uncertainty.

4. Restrictions on visits :

In order to limit the spread of the virus, visits were often restricted or even prohibited. This created communication challenges and reinforced the importance of digital means of maintaining the link between patients and their families.

5. Staff fatigue and stress:

Faced with constant pressure and increased workloads, FCRD staff often experienced physical and emotional fatigue. It was essential to put in place support and recognition measures for these front-line professionals.

6. Adaptability of care :

The rapid pace of discoveries concerning the virus and its implications has necessitated constant monitoring and regular updating of care protocols.

7. Logistical challenges:

Whether it's the supply of medicines, PPE or equipment, the FCRD supply chain has been put to the test.

8. Post-COVID rehabilitation:

The very nature of the disease, with its respiratory, cardiac and neurological complications, has necessitated a rethink of rehabilitation programmes. Post-COVID patients have specific needs that have required a tailored and often multidisciplinary approach.

The pandemic has undoubtedly transformed the FCRD landscape, highlighting the need for effective preparedness, cross-sector coordination and the ability to respond rapidly to changing situations. While the challenges have been many, they have also provided an opportunity to rethink and optimise the organisation and delivery of care for the future.

Adaptation and innovation
in response to the crisis.

The global health crisis has highlighted the ability of the medical sector, including Follow-up and Rehabilitation Care (FRC), to innovate and adapt rapidly to exceptional circumstances. The adaptations and innovations have been many and varied, ranging from practical changes to therapeutic approaches and technological solutions.

1. Telemedicine and tele-rehabilitation:
The pandemic accelerated the adoption of telemedicine, enabling professionals to continue monitoring patients without exposing them to the risk of infection. In addition, remote rehabilitation sessions have been set up for certain patients, using dedicated applications and platforms.

2. On-line training :
Faced with the need to train staff quickly on new procedures, COVID-19 protocols and care techniques, many institutions have developed online training modules, which are often permanently accessible.

3. Adoption of new technologies :
Tools such as symptom tracking applications, remote monitoring devices and UV disinfection robots have been integrated into FCRD routines to improve the safety and efficiency of care.

4. Revised care protocols:
Appropriate protocols for the management of post-COVID patients have been drawn up, taking into account the respiratory, cardiac and neurological complications associated with this disease.

5. Modular spaces:
Some FCRD have redesigned their spaces to create areas dedicated to patients with COVID-19, with optimised ventilation and air filtration.

6. Staff well-being programmes:
Aware of the psychological and emotional challenges their

teams have had to face, many establishments have set up support programmes, relaxation and meditation sessions, or dedicated rest areas.

7. Improved communication :

With visiting restrictions in place, communication between medical teams, patients and their families has become essential. Solutions, such as tablets for videoconferencing and regular updates via dedicated applications, have been developed.

8. Partnerships and collaboration :

Given the scale of the crisis, collaboration between hospitals, research centres, universities and industry has intensified to exchange knowledge, share resources and jointly develop solutions.

9. Participation in research :

Many FCRD have actively participated in COVID-19 research, particularly in post-infectious rehabilitation, contributing to the development of new guidelines and recommendations.

10. Planning and preparing for the future:

The pandemic highlighted the need for robust contingency planning. FCRD have therefore invested in training, updating emergency plans and stockpiling equipment.

While the crisis has presented unprecedented challenges, it has also catalysed a wave of innovations and adaptations that have not only helped to overcome the immediate difficulties, but have also laid the foundations for a more resilient healthcare system that is prepared for the future.

Lessons learned and implications for the future of the FCRD.

The pandemic has been an eye-opening period for the medical world, and in particular for Continuing Care and

Rehabilitation (CRH). Institutions have faced unprecedented challenges, but they have also learned valuable lessons that will have lasting implications for the future of FCRD.

1. System resilience :
FCRD have discovered their ability to adapt quickly by reconfiguring spaces, adopting modified protocols and pivoting to technological solutions. This ability to react quickly will be cultivated in the future to respond to potential crises.

2. Telemedicine is here to stay:
While telemedicine was adopted out of necessity during the pandemic, it has proved its effectiveness and is likely to be permanently integrated into FCRD practices, offering greater flexibility and accessibility for patients.

3. Importance of ongoing training:
The need for regular updating of staff knowledge and skills was highlighted. The CRDD will invest more in continuing education, using digital formats to facilitate access.

4. Interdisciplinary collaboration :
The complexity of managing COVID-19 patients has reinforced the importance of collaboration between different medical specialties. This collaborative approach is likely to be strengthened in the years ahead.

5. Reinforcement of hygiene protocols :
The strengthened hygiene protocols adopted during the pandemic will be maintained, ensuring better protection against a variety of infections, not just COVID-19.

6. Equipment and technologies :
The pandemic has accelerated the adoption of new technologies. These innovations, whether in the form of remote monitoring systems or communication platforms, will be permanently integrated into FCRD practices.

7. Emergency planning :
FCRD now recognises the importance of emergency preparedness and planning. Plans will be regularly updated

and tested to ensure that facilities are ready to respond quickly to any future crisis.

8. Patient-centred care :

The importance of communication and education of patients and their families has been highlighted. FCRD will strengthen their commitment to a patient-centred approach, emphasising patient education, communication and involvement in the care process.

9. Staff mental health:

The emotional challenges faced by staff during the pandemic have highlighted the importance of mental wellbeing. FCRD will place greater emphasis on psychological support for their staff.

10. Strategic intelligence :

The ability to keep up with rapidly evolving medical knowledge during a crisis will be built into regular FCRD practice, with a focus on research, technology watch and updating practice accordingly.

Although the pandemic has been a tumultuous time for the NHS, the lessons learned have created an opportunity for these institutions to renew, strengthen and prepare for a future where care will be more flexible, collaborative, technologically advanced and patient-centred.

Chapter 17:
PROFESSIONAL DEVELOPMENT AND FUTURE PROSPECTS

Specialisation opportunities and continuing education.

The world of Continuing Care and Rehabilitation (CCR) offers a wide range of opportunities for nurses wishing to specialise or enhance their skills. The complex and rapidly evolving nature of the medical field means that continuing education is not just a benefit, but a necessity. Here is a fluid overview of the specialisation and continuing education opportunities available to nurses in the FCRD field:

Rehabilitation medicine is a constantly evolving discipline, reflecting advances in medical science and the diversification of patient needs. So for nurses, adapting and specialising is not only an opportunity, but also an imperative if they are to provide the best possible quality of care.

1. Specialisations according to patient needs :
- **Paediatric FCRD:** Focusing on the care of children requires a particular understanding of their specific needs.
- **Geriatric FCRD:** The elderly, with their multiple pathologies and frailty, require a tailored approach.
- **Neurorehabilitation:** For patients with brain injuries or other neurological disorders, specific neurological skills are essential.
- **Cardiac rehabilitation:** Following major cardiovascular events, patients require specialised care to regain optimum quality of life.

2. Advanced care techniques :
- **Pain management:** Techniques are evolving rapidly, requiring regular training to provide the best possible care.
- **Mobilisation techniques:** Early and effective mobilisation is crucial to rehabilitation. Specialised training courses can further develop skills in this area.

3. Psychosocial skills :
- **Intercultural communication:** Understanding and respecting patients' cultural diversity is vital, and training courses can help to develop these skills.
- **Mental health:** Working with mental health professionals and identifying psychological problems in rehabilitation patients are specialist areas.

4. Management and leadership :
For those wishing to progress into management or leadership roles, training in care management, clinical leadership or administration may be beneficial.

5. Research and technology :
The world of FCRD is constantly benefiting from advances in technology and research. Nurses can specialise in the use of modern rehabilitation equipment, or even take part in clinical research to improve FCRD practices.

6. Medical ethics:
With issues as sensitive as end-of-life or treatment decisions, training in medical ethics can be invaluable.

The FCRD landscape is rich and varied, offering nurses a multitude of opportunities to develop, specialise and excel. By investing in continuing education, they can not only enrich their careers, but also improve the quality of care they provide to their patients.

Research in the FCRD: where are we going?

Research in post-acute and rehabilitation care (PACR) has made major strides over the last few decades, with a constant focus on improving practices, optimising patient outcomes and integrating new technologies and methodologies. Being intrinsically multidisciplinary, FCRD lends itself to exploration in a variety of research directions. Let's take a look at where FCRD research is heading and what the emerging trends are.

Research in the CRH has always focused on people. Every advance and every discovery is guided by a fundamental objective: to facilitate recovery, improve quality of life and ensure patient autonomy. But as our understanding of medicine deepens, the avenues of research multiply.

1. Cutting-edge technologies in rehabilitation: Telemedicine, exoskeletons, virtual and augmented reality are all areas of interest. These tools, once relegated to the realms of science fiction, are now at the heart of FCRD research programmes. What's in it for us? Offering more appropriate, less invasive and sometimes even fun solutions to help patients with their rehabilitation.

2. Neuroplasticity: The brain is still revealing all its secrets. Research into neuroplasticity - the ability of the nervous system to reconfigure itself - is opening the way to more targeted treatments for brain injuries and neurodegenerative diseases.

3. Holistic approaches: Research is increasingly recognising the importance of a holistic approach, integrating the physical, mental and social aspects. The impact of nutrition, psychology and even complementary therapies such as meditation or yoga is increasingly being studied in the context of FCRD.

4. Personalised care: With advances in genomics and personalised medicine, there is growing interest in rehabilitation protocols tailored to the genetic or biochemical specificities of each patient.

5. Efficiency and optimisation: Given the economic pressures on healthcare systems, a great deal of research is aimed at identifying the most efficient methods and techniques for achieving the best results in the shortest possible time.

6. Training and education: Research does not stop with patients. How can we best train tomorrow's professionals? What are the most effective teaching tools? These are crucial questions if we are to guarantee high-quality care over the long term.

7. Impact of the environment : Research is increasingly looking at the influence of the environment - both physical and social - on rehabilitation. What is the best way to design care environments? What is the impact of nature or art on recovery?

FCRD research is a fast-growing field, where medicine, technology and the human and social sciences meet. As our society evolves, rehabilitation needs become more diverse, and FCRD research must be at the cutting edge to meet these challenges.

The future of FCRD demographic and medical challenges.

Faced with an ageing population and the emergence of new pathologies and medical challenges, Continuing Care and Rehabilitation (CCR) is at a croFCRDoads. It is essential to anticipate and adapt to these changes in order to guarantee high-quality care and optimal patient management. In an ever-changing world, what are the major issues and future prospects for CRH in the face of demographic and medical challenges?

1. Demographics: an ageing population

Increasing life expectancy and an ageing population are one of the greatest challenges facing the FCRD sector. With age often come chronic illnesses, motor disabilities, neurological disorders and other conditions that require intensive rehabilitation. This means that FCRD have to be prepared to care for increasing numbers of elderly patients, who often have a wide range of specific needs.

2. The emergence of new diseases

In addition to the illnesses traditionally treated in the CRH, new pathologies, often linked to our modern lifestyles, are emerging. Musculoskeletal disorders linked to sedentary work, psychosomatic conditions and the consequences of chronic stress are all new challenges for CRH teams.

3. A holistic approach to rehabilitation

Faced with these challenges, FCRD are increasingly recognising the importance of comprehensive patient care. This involves close collaboration between professionals from different backgrounds (medical, paramedical, psychological) and particular attention to the patient's socio-familial environment.

4. Technology at the service of rehabilitation

The rapid development of medical technologies is opening up incredible opportunities for CRHs. Robotics, virtual reality, telemedicine... These innovations are helping to improve care, personalise treatment and optimise rehabilitation. However, they also require ongoing training for professionals and substantial investment.

5. Prevention as the watchword

Faced with the increase in chronic diseases, the FCRD has a crucial role to play in prevention. Therapeutic education, promotion of a healthy lifestyle and early screening are all ways of reducing the incidence of certain diseases and improving patients' quality of life.

6. An organisational and economic challenge

The increase in patient numbers and the growing complexity of care are posing major organisational challenges. It is crucial to rethink the models for financing, managing and organising FCRD in order to guarantee optimal care while keeping costs under control.

7. Training and research, the pillars of development

To stay at the cutting edge, CRHs need to invest in training their teams and in research. This means not only incorporating the latest medical advances, but also developing new methodologies, participating in clinical trials and adopting a continuous improvement approach.

While the challenges are many, they also offer great opportunities for the CRH. The future of rehabilitation will involve an integrated, innovative and patient-centred approach, enabling us to support each individual throughout his or her health journey, whatever their condition or needs.

Chapter 18:
TESTIMONIALS AND CASE STUDIES

Sharing experience
veteran nurses in FCRD.

Sharing experiences, in particular those of veteran nurses in Follow-up and Rehabilitation Care (FCRD), provides an incomparable wealth of information. These first-hand accounts illustrate the day-to-day reality of the profession, with its joys, sorrows, challenges and successes. Here is an outline of what a chapter dedicated to these accounts might look like.

At the heart of rehabilitation, there are many veteran nurses who have lived through the years, providing care and comfort to FCRD patients. Their experiences are windows into the soul of the profession.

Marie, 25 years old in an FCRD :
"I started young, with boundless energy. The FCRD was a new world for me, where each patient had a story to tell. I learned that beyond technical care, listening was essential. I remember Paul, a man in his fifties who suffered a stroke. His rehabilitation took a long time, but each step forward was a victory. These moments of shared joy are what fuel my passion.

Olivier, 30 years of service:
"CRDD has changed a lot. Technological developments have brought incredible tools. But what hasn't changed is the human relationship. When I started out, I was told that I was the link between the patient and the doctor. Today, I realise that I'm also the link between the patient and

themselves, helping them to rediscover themselves after a trauma or illness."

Fatima, 20 years at the bedside:
"Every patient is a world. In the FCRD, we see people at a very vulnerable time in their lives. They are often lost and frightened. Our role goes far beyond care. It's also about bringing hope. I'm thinking of Léa, a young woman who was in a road accident. She was convinced that she would never walk again. With time, care and a lot of encouragement, she took her first steps. You never forget moments like that.

Jean-Pierre, nurse then health executive, 35 years in an FCRD :
"Coordination is essential. You never work alone in FCRD. It's a team, and every member counts. Over the years, I've learnt to value every skill, whether medical, paramedical or administrative. Everything is linked, and a patient's successful rehabilitation is often the result of teamwork.

These testimonials illustrate the richness and complexity of work in the FCRD. They highlight the central role played by nurses, who are simultaneously carers, educators, coordinators and emotional supporters. They remind us that medicine is above all a human art, where each patient is unique and each story precious.

Analysis of real clinical cases and problem-solving.

The analysis of real-life clinical cases in FCRD offers a unique opportunity to gain a concrete understanding of the challenges and issues involved in rehabilitation. These case studies allow us to tackle complex situations and develop in-depth thinking about nursing interventions. Here is an exploration of one such case, with the resolution of the associated problems.

Clinical case: Mrs Dupont
Mrs Dupont, aged 67, was admitted to the FCRD following hip surgery. She has a history of hypertension and diabetes. Her daughter accompanied her and expressed concern about her mother's ability to regain her independence.

Problem 1: Post-operation pain
Nursing intervention: Regular assessment of Mrs Dupont's pain, administration of analgesics as prescribed, monitoring of side effects, patient education on pain management.
Problem 2: Risk of surgical site infection
Nursing intervention: Daily monitoring of the surgical wound, checking for signs of infection (redness, warmth, discharge), educating the patient about the importance of hygiene.
Problem 3: Anxiety in the patient and her daughter
Nurse's involvement: Creating a listening space for Mrs Dupont and her daughter, explaining the stages of rehabilitation, reassuring them about the skills of the care team, suggesting sessions with a psychologist if necessary.
Problem 4: Managing co-morbidities (hypertension, diabetes)
Nursing care: Regular monitoring of blood sugar levels and blood pressure, administration of prescribed medication, educating Mrs Dupont about the importance of a balanced diet and taking her medication regularly.

Problem 5: Rehabilitation and early mobilisation
Nursing involvement: Working closely with the physiotherapists, encouraging the patient to take an active part in the sessions, monitoring Mrs Dupont's tolerance of

the exercises, adjusting the sessions according to progress.

By analysing this clinical case, we can see that the FCRD nurse plays a central role in the overall care of the patient. They assess, intervene, educate and coordinate care to ensure the best possible quality of care. Each situation is unique, and interventions must be tailored to the specific needs of each patient. The analysis of clinical cases helps to develop a holistic vision of care, integrating medical, psychological, social and educational aspects.

The power of humanity in healing and rehabilitation.

The power of humanity in healing and rehabilitation is an essential element that is often underestimated in the modern medical world. Despite technological evolution and scientific advances, the human touch, attentive listening and compassion remain powerful tools in the healing process.

At the heart of this power lies the ability to create meaningful connections. For FCRD patients, rehabilitation is as much about the mind as the body. The physical challenges are obvious, but the emotional, psychological and spiritual challenges that accompany a long convalescence or chronic illness are just as real. Carers who adopt a humanistic approach see the patient as a whole, recognising their needs, hopes, fears and desires.

Encouraging words, a helping hand or simply a quiet presence at a time of pain or discouragement can be powerful catalysts for recovery. These gestures boost the patient's confidence and motivation to continue with the treatments, exercises and therapies needed for rehabilitation.

Humanity in care also enhances the well-being of care staff. By establishing genuine links with their patients, carers often find meaning and deep satisfaction in their work, which can protect them from burnout and burnout.

It is also in this humanity that families and loved ones find support. Witnessing the suffering of a loved one is an ordeal in itself. But seeing that person treated with dignity, respect and compassion can bring invaluable comfort.

As we live in an age of rapid medical innovation, it's crucial to remember that humanity is at the heart of healing. Machines can help diagnose, drugs can treat, but it is the human spirit, with its resilience, compassion and ability to connect, that is often the key to true healing and rehabilitation.

Conclusion:

The undeniable importance of the nurse in the FCRD.

The FCRD nurse is a central figure, an essential link in the complex process of rehabilitation and care. Their role goes beyond simple technical procedures or medical monitoring: they are the real link between the patient, their family and the medical team, ensuring consistency and continuity of care.

From the moment of admission, the nurse lays the foundations for a relationship of trust, which is crucial to a harmonious healing process. This trust is built not only on technical competence, but also on empathy, listening and the ability to reassure. In the delicate context of rehabilitation, where patients are often confronted with their own limitations, frustrations and fears, the nurse becomes a first-rate psychological support, a reassuring presence on a daily basis.

But its scope goes far beyond the emotional aspect. The nurse is also a true orchestra conductor, brilliantly coordinating the interventions of the various health professionals. They keep a close eye on things, ensuring that each stage of the care plan is properly followed and adapted if necessary, while maintaining fluid communication with the doctors, physiotherapists, occupational therapists and other specialists involved.

The versatility of FCRD nurses is also remarkable. From one minute to the next, they can go from an advanced care technique, to a discussion on therapeutic patient education, to coordinating a mobility workshop. This ability to adapt, to juggle different roles, makes him a cornerstone of the FCRD.

What's more, faced with the challenges posed by changes in society, technology and medicine, nurses in the CRH are constantly reinventing themselves. They are often at the cutting edge of innovation, constantly seeking to improve their practices, to train and to keep up to date, in order to offer patients the best possible care.

If the FCRD is a place of second chances, rebirth and renewal, it is largely thanks to the commitment, passion and determination of the nurses who work there. They are living proof that humanity, dedication and skill can work together to transform lives, and it is this undeniable importance that makes them essential pillars of the world of rehabilitation.

Encouragement and advice for those new to the business.

Becoming a nurse in the CRH is an exciting but demanding adventure, full of obstacles but also moments of profound gratification. For those new to the profession, determination, patience and passion are essential. Here is some encouragement and advice to guide your first steps:

- **Learning is continuous**: Understand that every day is an opportunity to learn. Medicine is constantly evolving, and so are treatment techniques. Be curious, ask questions, and don't be afraid to say you don't know.
- **Patience is your best ally**: Progress in rehabilitation can be slow and sometimes invisible. Celebrate every little victory, however small, and remember that every patient is unique.

116

- **Establish links** : The relationship with the patient is at the heart of rehabilitation. Take the time to listen, understand and build a relationship of trust.
- **Surround yourself with people**: Your colleagues will be a valuable source of support, encouragement and advice. Don't hesitate to ask for their help, share your doubts and learn from their experience.
- **Take care of yourself**: The emotional burden can be heavy in the FCRD. It is essential to recognise your limits, adopt self-care strategies and seek help if necessary. Your well-being is essential if you are to provide the best possible care.
- **Stay the course**: There will be difficult days, complex situations and moments of doubt. Remember why you chose this profession, the difference you can make to patients' lives, and let that passion be your guide.
- **Continuous training**: Ongoing training is essential to stay up to date and strengthen your skills. Take advantage of specialisation opportunities, workshops and conferences to broaden your horizons.
- **Seek out mentoring**: Finding a mentor, an experienced figure who can guide, advise and support you, can be invaluable in the early years of your career.
- **Communication is key**: develop your communication skills, not only with patients but also with the medical team. Clear and effective communication is essential to ensure the best possible care.
- **Believe in yourself**: Finally, remember that every day, through your actions, your skills and your humanity, you make a difference. You have the ability to bring comfort, guide healing and change lives.

Dear newcomers, your journey in the FCRD has just begun, and what an adventure it promises to be! Embrace each challenge with heart and determination, because the world of rehabilitation has so much to offer you. You are the future of the FCRD, and we believe in you.

Glossary of medical terms.

A glossary of medical terms is an essential addition to any book aimed at healthcare professionals, especially for novices. Although I cannot cover all the terms you might wish to include, here is a selection relevant to an FCRD context:

- **Analgesic**: Drug designed to reduce or eliminate pain.
- **Atrophy**: Reduction in the volume of a tissue, organ or part of the body, generally due to disease or lack of use.
- **Functional assessment**: Assessment of a person's abilities and limitations in various activities of daily living.
- **Cognition**: All the mental functions that include thinking, memory, judgement and problem-solving.
- **Decubitus**: Lying down. The term is often associated with ulcers that may develop as a result of prolonged pressure on a particular area of the body.
- **Occupational therapy**: Therapy using productive or creative activities to help regain or maintain maximum independence.
- **Physiotherapy:** Therapy using movement to treat and prevent certain conditions.
- **Passive mobility**: Movement of a part of the body without any active effort on the part of the patient, generally carried out by a therapist or an appliance.
- **Neurodegenerative**: Refers to diseases characterised by the progressive degradation of nerve cells or neurons.
- **Orthosis**: External appliance or device used to correct or alleviate a deformity or dysfunction.
- **Palliative**: Treatment designed to relieve symptoms without treating the underlying cause of the disease.

- **Rehabilitation**: The process of helping a person to regain or improve their functional abilities following an illness or injury.
- **Sequela**: A consequence of an illness or injury that persists after the initial cause has been treated or cured.
- **Spasticity**: An increase in muscle tone that can lead to spasms or involuntary muscle contractions.
- **Deep vein thrombosis (DVT)**: formation of a blood clot in a deep vein, usually in the leg.
- **Mechanical   ventilation**: Use of a machine to help a person breathe when they are unable to do so themselves.

Obviously, it would be necessary to add to this glossary in line with the topics covered throughout the book. The terms listed here are only an outline, but they provide a solid basis to help novices understand some of the specialist terms they may encounter in FCRD.

Additional resources
for training
and professional development.

Training and professional development are essential for any nurse wishing to keep abreast of the latest medical and technical advances and best practice. Here is a list of resources that FCRD nurses may find useful for their training and development:

- Professional associations :
    - *Ordre National des Infirmiers*: Offers training opportunities, events and resources for nurses.
    - *Association Française de Soins de Suite et de Réadaptation (AFFCRD) (French Association for Continuing Care and Rehabilitation):* specifically for CRH professionals, it offers training courses, conferences and workshops.
- Specialist newspapers and magazines:
    - *Revue de l'infirmière:* articles, case studies, research and news specific to the profession.
    - *Rehabilitation Care*: Focusing specifically on rehabilitation care, this journal covers new techniques, case studies and research.
- Online training :
    - Platforms such as *Coursera*, *Udemy* and *Khan Academy* offer courses on a variety of medical subjects, including rehabilitation.
- Conferences and workshops :
    - Participating in national and international events on rehabilitation care, general medicine and other related specialities.
- Books and manuals :
    - There are many books on specialist nursing care, rehabilitation, physiology and other

relevant subjects. It is advisable to consult new publications regularly.
- Professional social networks :
    - Platforms such as *LinkedIn make it* possible to join groups dedicated to rehabilitation care, where members share resources, studies and experiences.
- Mentoring programmes :
    - Look for mentoring opportunities, where experienced nurses guide and advise those new to the profession.
- Clinical research :
    - Keeping abreast of the latest research in the field of FCRD enables the latest findings to be incorporated into daily practice.
- Universities and training establishments :
    - Many of them offer continuing education courses, university diplomas or specialist certificates.
- Internships and rotations :
    - Think about doing work placements in different departments or establishments to gain diverse experience and complementary skills.

The medical world is constantly evolving, and it is crucial for healthcare professionals to continue to learn and develop throughout their careers. These resources, combined with a willingness to learn, can help nurses provide exceptional care to their patients and grow in their profession.

Useful links
and professional associations.

In the field of Continuing Care and Rehabilitation (CCR) and more broadly in the nursing sector, there are many professional associations and online resources that can offer support, information and continuing education opportunities to nurses. Here is a non-exhaustive list of useful links and professional associations:

- National professional associations :
    - **Ordre National des Infirmiers (ONI)**: The ONI is the official organisation representing nurses in France. It offers regulatory information, training opportunities and professional news.
    - ONI website
    - **Association Française de Soins de Suite et de Réadaptation (AFFCRD)**: This association focuses specifically on the issues and needs of professionals working in FCRD.
    - **Fédération Nationale des Infirmiers (FNI)**: This is one of the main trade unions representing self-employed nurses in France.
    - FNI website
- Other relevant associations :
    - **Association Française des Infirmiers(e)s de Rééducation et de Réadaptation (AFIRR)**: This association is dedicated to training, research and defending the professional interests of nurses working in re-education and rehabilitation.
    - **Association Nationale Française des Infirmiers et Infirmières Diplôm(e)s et Étudiants (ANFIIDE)**: ANFIIDE focuses on the

education, research and professional practice of nurses in France.

- ANFIIDE website

- Online resources :
  - **Infirmiers.com: This is** an information-rich web portal offering news, articles, discussion forums and resources for nurses.
    - Infirmiers.com website
  - **ActuSoins**: Online magazine devoted to nursing news.
    - ActuSoins website
  - **L'Infirmière Magazine**: A magazine for nursing professionals featuring articles, reports and case studies.
    - L'Infirmière Magazine

- International organisations :
  - **International Council of Nurses (ICN)**: Based in Geneva, this organisation works to ensure quality nursing care for all, foster economic development and promote women's rights.
    - CII website

- Training platforms :
  - **DPC (Continuing Professional Development)** : Official platform for continuing education for healthcare professionals, including nurses.
    - CPD website

- Forums and discussion groups :
  - Numerous online forums, such as those on Infirmiers.com and other specialist platforms, allow nurses to exchange experiences, advice and information on a variety of subjects.

These associations and resources can help nurses stay informed, develop their skills and connect with their peers. It's a good idea to sign up to their newsletters or follow them on social networks to keep up to date with the latest news and opportunities.

www.ingramcontent.com/pod-product-compliance
Lightning Source LLC
Chambersburg PA
CBHW062325290526
45794CB00005B/1902